Praise for *The Citizen Patient*

"A tour de force. Compelling and extremely well-informed.
Hadler offers important new insights."
—MARK HALL, professor of law and public health,
Wake Forest University

"Blending best science, sound ethics, compassionate clinical care,
and economic realism, Hadler exhorts patients to take control of their own
health and health system to save the United States from fiscal disaster."
—GEORGE D. LUNDBERG, M.D., former editor in chief (1982–99),
Journal of the American Medical Association

"Sweeping in scope. Dr. Hadler's prescription for reform is radical and
compassionate and could dramatically improve the health of every citizen
while simultaneously saving vast sums of money."
—JEANNE LENZER, medical investigative journalist

"An informed critique and evaluation of the current U.S. health-care system
with creative suggestions as to how it can be restructured for the benefit of
patients. Hadler's views are always interesting, original, and provocative."
—ARTHUR RUBENSTEIN, M.D., Perelman School of Medicine,
University of Pennsylvania

"Doctors should read this book and examine their motives and
their consciences. Anyone who thinks they might ever become a patient
should also use it to understand the hidden agendas at work in
medicine—which might not necessarily be in their best interests!"
—LOIS ROGERS, international health-care commentator,
former *Sunday Times London* health and social affairs editor

"Dr. Hadler illuminates the inconvenient truths that prevent real
reform and offers bold new directions. He pulls back the veil to reveal
the ignorance that surrounds most modern concepts of health care
and disease, shows that our efforts—in both time and dollars—have
been misguided, and offers an alternative path that is simple and
at odds with conventional thinking."
—LARRY VAN HORN, associate professor of economics and
management, Vanderbilt University

The Citizen Patient

The
Citizen Patient

Reforming Health Care for the Sake of the Patient,

Not the System

Nortin M. Hadler, M.D.

THE UNIVERSITY OF NORTH CAROLINA PRESS | CHAPEL HILL

This book was published with the assistance of the
H. EUGENE AND LILLIAN YOUNGS LEHMAN FUND
of the University of North Carolina Press.
A complete list of books published in the Lehman Series
appears at the end of the book.

Set in Utopia by Tseng Information Systems, Inc.
Manufactured in the United States of America
The paper in this book meets the guidelines for permanence
and durability of the Committee on Production Guidelines for
Book Longevity of the Council on Library Resources.
The University of North Carolina Press has been a member of
the Green Press Initiative since 2003.

Library of Congress Cataloging-in-Publication Data
Hadler, Nortin M.
The citizen patient : reforming health care for the sake of the patient,
not the system / Nortin M. Hadler. — 1st ed.
p. ; cm.
Includes bibliographical references and index.
ISBN 978-1-4696-0704-7 (cloth : alk. paper)
I. Title.
[DNLM: 1. Delivery of Health Care—United States.
2. Health Care Reform—United States. 3. Patient Participation—United States.
4. Physician-Patient Relations—United States. W 84 AA1]
362.10973—dc23
2012041236

17 16 15 14 13   5 4 3 2 1

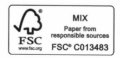

For Carol S. Hadler, *always*

Contents

Figures and Tables

Acknowledgments

I am privileged to work in one of America's underground academic clinical departments, of which there are many more across the country. Here, committed clinicians, clinical scholars, and clinical investigators hang out. Most keep their heads down, engaged in their life pursuits with determination and enjoying the self-satisfaction of ever-improving competence. None seek rewards or career options that veer away from these pursuits or that might possibly corrupt their professionalism. These men and women were once the essence of American medicine. Today, they are a threatened species. I am proud and grateful to be one in this fold. This is my peer group, without whose acceptance and encouragement the writing of *The Citizen Patient* would have been a burden instead of a mission. Perhaps *The Citizen Patient* will rally others to the mission of these professionals. Until then, they might find comfort in these words by e. e. cummings:

> To be nobody but yourself in a
> world which is doing its best day
> and night to make you like
> everybody else means to fight the
> hardest battle which any human
> being can fight and never stop
> fighting.

And I am fortunate and privileged to have found an author's home at the University of North Carolina Press. It is truly a home with a family that has supported my efforts through four books, culminating in *The Citizen Patient*. I owe particular thanks to "my" editors, David Perry (editor in chief of the Press) and Jay Mazzocchi. David has worked tirelessly to aim me toward the goal of clarity, and Jay has added the polish. I thank Gina Mahalek and Dino Battista and their colleagues for working to make sure the products of all these efforts see the light of day.

The Citizen Patient

Introduction

There is a difference between the health of the person and the health of the people. My last four books dissect the former from the perspective of the patient. *The Last Well Person* (2004), *Worried Sick* (2008), *Stabbed in the Back* (2009), and *Rethinking Aging* (2011) are meant to teach readers how to ask "Will this really benefit me?" when faced with prescriptions for improving or preserving their health. Those who have read these books are in a position to recognize medicalization and overtreatment in all phases of life and for myriad complaints; furthermore, they will understand what is entailed in making informed decisions about their own medical care.

The Citizen Patient does not further dissect the patient-physician relationship solely to enlighten individual medical decision making. Rather, it unpacks and examines the modern doctor-patient relationship—and the many perversities that characterize the American "health-care system"—in order to enable readers, as enlightened Citizen Patients, to put that knowledge in the service of change.

A necessary first step in devising a rational solution to our national health-care problem is preparing all patients to take responsibility for assuring that whatever is being said or offered or done will really be to their benefit. If "health care" and the system that underpins it were intrinsically trustworthy, patients could relax, secure in the knowledge that whatever happens to them has a salutary benefit-to-risk ratio. Sadly, we know that this is not the case; in fact, the present health-care system is structured to frustrate that security.

Any discussion of "health care" must necessarily begin with a discussion of "health." What do we mean by "health"? One can enjoy "good" health or suffer "bad" health. Is "bad" health no more than the absence of "good" health? Is there a continuum between "good" and "bad" health? Can either be objectified reliably?

Good health is not the absence of symptoms; all of us will suffer symptoms repeatedly, symptoms that give us pause without compromising our belief that we are basically well. Episodes of backache, headache, heartache, "colds," "flu," and much more are predicaments of life for which most of us are a match most of the time. Despite such predicaments, we can remain in good health.

Nor is health the absence of disease. If we define disease as pathology, as abnormalities in our anatomy or physiology, by midlife all of us harbor diseases—and I mean important diseases. Some of these are so commonplace as to be part of the course of life: gray hair, bunions, degenerative changes in the spine, hardening of the arteries, some forms of cancer, and the like. Some are lying in wait to smite our good health. Some are contenders for the ultimate smiting, the cause of our demise. Most will still be lying in wait on that fateful day. Despite our diseases, we can remain in good health.

Health is not a purely scientific construct; the components of health that can be quantified and studied systematically barely scratch the surface of what most of us mean by good health. Science is no match for individual perceptions of well-being, for the temporal component of well-being, or for the vagaries of the social construction of well-being. A century ago, obesity indicated good health, while today it's generally considered to indicate bad health, even though we know that it is the correlative socioeconomic status that influences health far more than heftiness itself. A century ago, orgasms were considered bad for you; today, their absence is considered something that merits treatment.

Health in general, and good health in particular, does not lend itself readily to easy understanding because it has many components and reflects so much that is our humanity. In that regard, it is similar to other hard-to-define concepts, such as "love" and "job satisfaction." Many elements contribute to health, only some of which are defined and all of which display enormous individuality.

That being the case, what do we mean by "health care," the "health-care system," and "health-care reform"? These and many similar terms are no longer the language of policy; they have become common parlance. They all presume that good health will result if we prevent bad health. Further, if "bad" health surmounts our defenses, we can call on trained professionals whose job it is to identify and try to fix the diseases and disorders that render health "bad" so that "good" health will reemerge. I am a man of this cloth. I am trained, experienced, and committed to this strategy. I am also convinced that this strategy encompasses but a small component of health care, and an exclusive focus on it perverts the health-care system and diverts the goal of rational health-care reform. I am writing this book to recruit the reader to this expansive, perhaps radical, and certainly iconoclastic view.

This is not to say that a strategy of prevent-treat-cure is worthless. To the contrary, it is my life's work. It is what we think of when we exalt "medicine." However, it is a strategy that demands an exquisite moral compass. It is a strategy that must have no agenda other than to benefit the individual patient. If the *process* that serves the strategy becomes the goal, the patient is placed at risk of becoming the excuse rather than the beneficiary. The more the process is valued and rewarded for its own sake, the greater the personal price paid by the patient. I argue that this dialectic is approaching the extreme in America and thereby setting precedents around the globe.

This is a counterintuitive argument in a country wont to flaunt its medicine as the "best in the world." It becomes a compelling argument when one critically examines the process from the perspective of the patient enmeshed in the health-care system, not from the perspective of the system that promulgates the process.

In this book, I am enlisting you, whether you are a patient or not, in the larger project of changing the central question from "What's good for me?" to "What's the best way to organize health care so that I can have more confidence it will deliver what's good for me?" In order to facilitate this transition in mindset, chapters 1 through 6 present different perverse aspects of American health care as an object lesson. I chose these six aspects not only because they are harmful but also because they are quite amenable to reform once they are recognized for what they are. They are not ordered in importance. Chapter 7 sets forth a different approach to assuring health and insuring disease that would result if we were to take advantage of the knowledge gained in the six object lessons. We would have a rational health-care system that knew no other master than the health and welfare of the citizenry. In the final chapter, I return to the primary encounter in health care—the doctor-patient encounter in the clinic—and the possibility that it could once again become the site of a collaborative relationship between partners. We would all be advantaged by access to the caring environment discussed in that chapter.

1

Shills

WHEN PROFIT TRUMPS BENEFIT

Health care in the United States is ethically compromised. About that, there is no debate. The debate is over the *degree* of compromise and the even-more-heated question of what to do about it. The Institute of Medicine and nearly every other professional organization in the health arena have chimed in. The areas examined include medical errors, ethnic and racial disparities in provision of care, uneven quality of care, antiquated record keeping, and administrative inefficiency. They talk about overdiagnosis, overtreatment, and overhead. Each of these areas is surrounded by clouds of obfuscation, a predictable result of all the finger pointing. Hiding in the clouds is an essence that renders the U.S. health-care system essentially ethically bankrupt. That essence is conflict of interest.

A goodly percentage of the wealth of the country, approaching 20 percent of the gross domestic product each year, is commandeered by the health-care system. In chapter 2, we examine the health expenditures and healthfulness of many countries in the resource-advantaged world. Yet the United States gets the least "bang" despite expending the most "buck." Most of the monies expended in the United States—at least half of this largesse—pass through the system into the pockets of "stakeholders" without advantaging a *single* patient. The per capita expenditure of every other resource-advantaged country is half that of the United States or less without disadvantaging their patients by even an iota. In the United

States, the "system" and its myriad stakeholders are no longer the infra-structure; they are the *raison d'être*. Furthermore, the marketing, lobby-ing, and pandering is so well funded that entire institutions have been co-opted. Congress tilts toward the status quo thanks to the efforts of legions of lobbyists, as many as six per member of Congress. Medical education is now a "loss center" barely discernible in "academic health centers," which are barely academic and consider health care no more than a profit center. Regulatory agencies are often handmaidens of a political agenda or of powerful outside influences. The list goes on and depressingly on.

There is a desperate need for a voice on Capitol Hill or in the White House demanding that the health-care system claim the moral high ground. A demonstrable benefit for patients must trump any demon-strable benefit for any other stakeholder. If an intervention has been studied and can't be shown to offer a meaningful benefit, it does not mat-ter how efficiently or expertly or profitably it is accomplished; it should not be done. Any voice calling for that kind of change will be quickly stifled by those with vested interests in the marginally useful and the use-less, unless Citizen Patients take up the cause.

The Disclosure Dodge in the Clinic

Arrangements between individual practitioners and drug or device pur-veyors are a rich source of conflict of interest. Academic health centers and unaffiliated hospitals are racing to write or expand policy statements on conflicts of interest that relate to the clinical activities of individual practitioners. Several in Congress, Senator Chuck Grassley (R) of Iowa for one, are investigating and legislating. Policy is targeting marketing methods that seem on the surface to be innocuous: the on-site "detail-ing" by drug and device representatives, the trinkets and "free meals," the samples that cause a physician to become more familiar with prescribing the product than with the product's limitations, the sponsored educa-tional programs that engender comfort with the sales personnel if not the product, and other tactics. All of these are easy targets for those putting forth policies that treat the collective conscience of my profession. That's overdue. So, too, is a peer review that examines the feigned or real naïveté on the part of professionals who claim they are above being influenced in such an obvious way. But physicians owe their patients much more. The fact that policy rather than personal ethics is necessary to bring an end to these obvious marketing schemes is a reproach to my profession.

"Detailing" is the pharmaceutical industry's euphemism for marketing to physicians at the site of their practice. Great numbers of young, educated men and women are recruited to this task because they are attractive and articulate and likely to be found so by practitioners. They are schooled in presenting the clinical pharmacology of their wares in the most favorable light. They are not to overstep the boundaries defined by the Food and Drug Administration (FDA) for the use of any of their wares, but they typically learn how to tiptoe along the limits. If they are caught crossing that line, their company faces fines and bad press, which some pharmaceutical firms have managed to overcome in a number of notorious examples, such as in the marketing of particular "pain pills." The detailing representatives ("reps") show up in offices and clinics and ask for signed permission to stock a medicine cabinet with samples. They make appointments with the practitioners to ply them with the "details" that should convince the practitioner of the value of their product. By default, detailing may be the practitioner's only exposure to the relevant clinical science since independently seeking such information is time-consuming and, for many, less appealing than a discussion with an attractive sales representative at the office or over lunch. Because of the inherent bias in such information, direct marketing to practitioners has been banished from many institutions, though not all. Those that have not denied access are likely to be swamped with free lunches and smiling sales representatives, with their bags full of samples, trinkets, and other gifts; and even though these representatives are banned from many institutions, private practices often remain open to them. Detailing to health-care professionals remains a leading expenditure in the pharmaceutical industry's marketing budget (Figure 1).

There is much more that affronts moral philosophy, much that is not as concrete as a drug sample or a pen with a logo. I am saddened to have to write this chapter. But this is an era in medicine when ethical failing is not idiosyncratic. We are not talking about the occasional rotten apple; we are talking about blight on the crop. Shouldn't we expect, at a minimum, that our physician disclose all real and potential conflicts of interest that might have a bearing on his or her clinical judgment? The disclosure of potential conflicts of interest at least assures patients that their physician is cognizant of biases that might compromise care, and some might find that reassuring.

I would go further, however. For me, the very need to disclose a potential conflict of interest signifies immorality. Convictions of right and wrong are emotion laden. If I do something I find morally wrong, I feel shame or guilt. If you do something I find morally wrong, my sentiment of

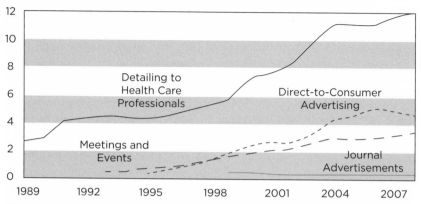

Figure 1. Promotional spending by type of marketing activity, 1989 to 2008 (in billions of dollars). The Congressional Budget Office (CBO) issued an "Economic and Budget Issue Brief" on December 2, 2009, regarding "Promotional Spending for Prescription Drugs." These data were obtained from SDI, a company that collects and sells information about the pharmaceutical industry. The SDI data set is not all-inclusive. However, the trends in the different categories are telling.

disapprobation is equally visceral, ranging from disappointment to out-rage. Let me be clear: there is an important distinction between moral judgments and conventional judgments. Guidelines for acceptable con-flicts of interest are an exercise in conventional judgment, about which I can countenance debate. However, the following syllogism expresses my moral judgment.

- No physician should knowingly enter into any arrangement that might compromise trustworthiness in any treatment act.
- Any physician who does not share this moral judgment is a compromised healer.

Given my stringent, intensely personal sentiment, it has been decades since I have acquiesced to being "detailed" by pharmaceutical represen-tatives, let alone allowing "samples" to be part of my practice. The hard-ware sales force has limited interest in this rheumatologist, and I have none in them. I shun all sorts of "freebies," and I have no interest in par-ticipating in any industry-supported educational undertaking where my participation might promote a hidden agenda on the part of the sponsor. In my practice, I have no conflicts to declare and no need to declare their absence. Furthermore, there is no need for any physician who shares my moral judgment to declare a conflict of interest. The absence of such is a given.

The seeds of these particular moral judgments were planted in my youth by my father as I accompanied him on house calls, and they germinated when I worked in proprietary hospitals half a century ago. I have had lapses, and I have been fooled on occasion. But these moral judgments have accompanied me on every patient contact for forty-five years.

Are they anachronistic? Am I a Luddite?

Medicine is no longer a cottage industry; it is a complex industrial enterprise. Medicine's front line, whatever it is called and whoever embodies it, is blurred. Physicians march to many drums, many of which demand a degree of fiscal savvy if not the occasional quick step. Could one argue that the modern physician is a match for whatever marketing biases might distort the message of pharmaceutical "detailing" and for agendas that might slant other educational events? Whose prescribing habits are influenced by the convenience and putative beneficence of drug samples, let alone by participation in flawed drug trials or marketing exercises masquerading as drug trials? What physician's clinical perspective can be bought with pizzas or trips to Monte Carlo? Isn't it insulting to suggest such? And doesn't the implication that the accompanying gifts and other largesse are forms of bribery aggravate the insult?

Of course it does. And so it should. In 2005 Minnesota officially limited pharmaceutical gifts to $50 per physician per year, effectively eliminating lunches and much else, including whatever physicians found appealing about meeting with pharmaceutical sales representatives and going to sponsored programs. The Massachusetts legislature banned direct marketing of pharmaceuticals and devices to providers. (The state can't touch direct-to-consumer advertising since the U.S. Supreme Court deemed it an example of freedom of speech.) However, the Massachusetts legislature is thinking about rescinding the ban because of pressure from Massachusetts's businesses, which claim to have suffered because medical conventions and other medical-marketing venues have found other states more accommodating.

Is this much ado about very little? Not to my way of thinking. Disclosure by the practitioner is nothing but a symptom of the pernicious ethos we will examine in greater detail shortly. The profession I love has been enveloped in a cloud of conflicting interests. The opinions of "thought leaders" are valued and rewarded by the purveyors advantaged by these opinions. Surgeons and other interventionalists are similarly rewarded by purveyors of the widgets and gizmos these physicians are wont to advocate. Professional societies appear more and more like industry subsidiaries and professional meetings more and more like market days. "Academic health centers" and similar large medical institutions seem more interested in "throughput" and supping at the "translational research" troughs than in valuing bedside excellence. And all this is sanctioned, even applauded, by oversight bodies. The FDA has no constraints on the consultancies of advisers, medical journals find "declarations" of conflictual relationships to be cleansing, academic health centers bid for drug trials to fuel their "translational" profit centers, and interventionalists are coddled if they regale the uninitiated with their technological prowess. The ethos is so entrenched that even the patients of spine surgeons see no problem if they are offered a device purveyed by a manufacturer for whom their surgeon is a paid consultant.

Well, I see a problem for which no degree of disclosure is a match. The only match is for the members of my profession to learn to wear, with pride, the moral judgments I detailed above and to decry the behavior of any physician not so inclined. Disclosure should not seem necessary, and it is never sufficient. For the Citizen Patient, it is a red flag.

The Disclosure Dodge in the Medical Literature

"Industry" is not a curse word. Industry is the fountainhead of jobs that sustain and nurture all of us directly or indirectly. Furthermore, relationships between industry personnel and professionals not employed by industry are not necessarily wrong, let alone evil. To the contrary, such relationships can enhance the productivity of both parties. The challenge for the independent professional, whether based in the academy or not, is to guarantee that the relationship does not distort or compromise that professional's primary role as educator, physician, therapist, clergy, or whatever.

On what can one base such a guarantee? In medicine, the professional is recruited to the task by an industry that seeks to be advantaged by that professional's expertise and is willing to reward the professional with influence, money, or other barter. The professional is always marching to two drums, one that beats for industrial success and another that beats for the benefit of the patients who are the primary responsibility. I am willing to call a halt to such arrangements whenever there is the possibility that marching to industry's drum can compromise the care of the patient or the education of those involved in that care.

That is not the consensus today, nor is it common practice. The consensus is that judgment regarding any compromise should be passed on to the interested observer—the reader, the audience, the grant reviewer, and the like. This is accomplished by disclosing the potentially compromising relationship on institutional forms, during public presentations, and as appendages to any professional publications. Many publications, particularly those that involve pharmaceuticals and medical devices, have long lists at the end detailing potential conflictual arrangements of the authors, such as paid consultancies, grants from purveyors, and equity positions. Among such authors, there seems to be a certain pride when one's list is longer than another's.

How about all the editorialists? Journal editors invite physicians to write editorials designed to put a particular research paper into a broader context than the authors do in the discussion of their results. The editorialists are chosen because they are respected for their contributions to this particular research area and because they can be counted on to say something interesting. I can tell you from many such experiences that it is a challenge to find an appropriate footing between destructively critical, excessively exuberant, and unnecessarily self-referential. It is the last tendency that represents my conflictual challenge, since I have done all I can to eschew formal external conflictual relationships. What about the editorialist who has more than purely intellectual conflicts of interest lurking between the lines? Is disclosure of financial and other entanglements enough to enable the reader to accept the editorial as a sage guide to the research under consideration? The editorial board of one prominent journal, the *New England Journal of Medicine*, thought not. But then they went on to the absurdity of quantifying in monetary terms the degree to which conflictual relationships might compromise sagacity. If the editorialist was compensated more than $10,000 in any given year by any entity the editorialist deems relevant, recusal should follow. The editorial board argued that there had to be some leeway or they would have difficulty identifying any nonconflicted editorialists. This argument is in keeping with policy statements by the National Institutes of Health and the American Association of Medical Colleges. I find it a reproach at so many levels, not the least of which is to the principle of peer review. It suggests that peer review is for sale, and it is relatively cheap.

Is anyone reassured by all this disclosing? I am not. To the contrary, I look askance at disclosers and at the substance that is being put forth in editorials or research papers by these compromised authors. And I look askance when clinical investigators disclose financial arrangements with for-profit enterprises that contract them to study the benefits patients might derive from their products. I am not surprised when study after study documents that when the assessment of a drug or device is industry supported, the result is far more likely to be positive than when the assessment of the same drug or device is government supported. I am not surprised by studies that demonstrate similar bias when an editorialist has some financial arrangement with the topic of the editorial. Disclosure be damned; give me uncompromising ethical behavior.

But that doesn't mean that the divide between industry and nonindustry scientists is inviolate. If professionals based in industry and professionals based in governmental or nonprofit organizations feel the need to interact at a professional level, there are venues that are meant to foster such interchange, including professional meetings and publications. Many a "blockbuster" drug has been developed because industry scientists took advantage of openly disseminated insights that were generated by nonindustry scientists supported by governmental research grants. One might wonder about the equity of a system in which the taxpayer contributes both to the pharmaceutical firm's profit margin and development costs. But the interchange itself is a testimony to the ethical nature of the scientific process, an ethic that values peer review and transparency. Neither peer review nor transparency—transparency in particular—comes naturally. In both the private and public arenas, transparency is usually restrained and peer review often distorted by the competitive nature of scientific practice. The desire to be the first to do something is ingrained. Primacy is certified in the private sector by patent or licensure and rewarded by a competitive advantage in the marketplace. In the public sector, primacy is certified by publication and rewarded by recognition and advancement. All scientists guard their intellectual property to some extent until primacy is certified.

Conflicts of interest arise whenever this dynamic falls victim to greed. Science at its purest hones its methods and bridles its interpretations to disprove any hypothesis that interests the scientist undertaking the experiment, including hypotheses that can lead to marketable and profitable outcomes. This is a fragile ethic that is always victimized by any relationship that places profit above refutationist science. Professionals of stature are also people, often very ambitious people. Achieving monetary gains and achieving intellectual gains need not be dissonant. But if they cannot establish and maintain ethical boundaries, we all suffer the consequences.

The Institutionalization of Conflict of Interest

Disclosure extends beyond the individual level. The American Association of Medical Colleges undertook a national survey of medical school department chairs. The results were published in the *Journal of the Ameri-*

can *Medical Association* a couple of years ago. Almost two-thirds of those surveyed had a personal relationship with industry as a consultant, a board member, a paid speaker, or the like. The survey also asked about the sources of income for their departments. About one in five clinical departments enjoyed moneys for equipment and unrestricted funds, one in three received support for trainees, and the majority received support for "continuing medical education." Interestingly, the department chairs themselves felt that the more a chair was involved with industry, the less able the department was to "conduct independent unbiased research."

This is not just going on at the department level. It's also happening at the institutional level, where the largesse of industry can buy everything from the emphasis of a new or old department's research to the name of the school. My queasiness peaks when I know that the "CEO" of a large state-supported academic health center was also well compensated for sitting on the board of Medco, which at the time happened to be the pharmaceutical benefits manager for that state's employee health plan.

The American Hospital Business

At the start of the twentieth century, the American hospital had barely shed its vestiges as an almshouse. It was a charity institution dominated by charitable, even philanthropic, lay leaders. Those who could afford home-based care avoided hospitalization at all cost. This was to change through the century and dramatically after World War II. By the 1980s, the eminent Harvard historian Charles E. Rosenberg could write:

> The evolution of the hospital has reflected a clear and consistently understood vision. That vision looked inward towards the needs and priorities of the medical profession, inward toward the administrative and financial needs of the individual hospital, inward toward the body as a mechanism opaque to all but those with medical training—and away from that of patient as a social being and family member. It was a vision, moreover, so deeply felt as to preclude conscious planning, replacing it instead with a series of seemingly necessary actions. (*The Care of Strangers: The Rise of America's Hospital System* [1987])

Barely a vestige of this physician-dominated, inward-looking American hospital can be found in the current American hospital. I do not mourn for its loss. However, I do not applaud the American hospital that has replaced it. For example, my hospital was built with state funds and opened in the 1950s as North Carolina Memorial Hospital. For decades, a sign at the curb proudly declared that it was built "by and for the people of North Carolina." Today it is a complex of many buildings collectively called UNC Hospitals, largely built with monies generated by floating tax-free municipal bonds—an indebtedness that is serviced by hospital revenues. Furthermore, many of our buildings are off-site, satellites designed to recruit patients into our system before some other system captures them. As is true of all academic health centers and major nonacademic health centers, our administration has grown from a paltry few to buildings full of well-paid executives and their burgeoning staffs (Figure 2).

And our mission? Well, here's a recent announcement from our chief bureaucrat, who bears many titles, including CEO of UNC Hospitals and dean of the UNC School of Medicine:

> With the Board's approval, we can now move into implementation of the Strategic Market Plan. The same internal teams that helped us develop these plans will initiate the "Just Do It" phase, with those ideas we can put in place instantly without additional capacity. We have retained some of the consultants from Boston Consulting Group to work with [the] . . . VP, Operational Efficiency and Business Development to help us immediately focus on inpatient capacity. Next, we will focus on the pieces of the plan requiring capital expense and expansion. Finally, there are some areas of the strategic plan that require significant organizational change.
>
> The next steps toward implementing the newly approved strategic plan involve optimizing efficiency and utilization in the 13 service lines while also improving relationships with outside organizations that partner with us to care for our patients. With the help of our 13 teams, we will now move forward with implementation, developing budgets and estimating timelines. This is an aggressive growth plan, the success of which will depend on continuously improving our quality and efficiency.

Charles Rosenberg's description of the American hospital and the strategic market plan above were penned only twenty-five years apart. The mind is boggled both by the rapidity of the transition and by its attendant cognitive dissonance.

Some of Rosenberg's conclusions about the vision of the twentieth-century hospital pertain to its twenty-first-century successor. Both look "away from that of patient as a social being and family member." And for both, the *raison d'être* is "so deeply felt as to preclude conscious planning, replacing it instead with a series of seemingly necessary actions."

The striking difference is that today's vision is far more appropriate for a multisite, profit-generating retail enterprise than any notion a Citizen Patient might imagine for a hospital. A retail enterprise, though, is at risk of bankruptcy if it is mismanaged—the fate of a Kmart or a Sears. But the modern hospital complex has come into being because there has been no such accountability. Rather, there is unbridled greed at the public's expense. There is also little transparency, which is why the Citizen Patient is so befuddled. The public has accepted as fact that costliness reflects quality and complexity of care and that the "best" hospital deserves the most money. This bears witness to the old adage about fooling all of the people some of the time. Perhaps a peek at examples of the nitty-gritty of health-care expenditures and the ways these institutions set their spending priorities will convince you of the need to demand transparency about the outside organizations that partner with hospitals and about the financial structure of the hospital itself.

FACILITY FEES

Would you go to Walmart if they charged you an entry fee to cover their administrative costs? That cost is built into their pricing structure for the goods they sell. And you might be sorely tempted to go elsewhere if that other place charged less for comparable goods. Pricing of comparable goods was the secret to Walmart's success. Private-sector American medicine has always operated on this model; you or your insurer were charged for services with the understanding that the services were priced so as to cover overhead. Without fanfare, however, American hospitals and clinics have introduced "facility fees." These fees vary from the significant to the outrageous. There have been lawsuits, including class-action lawsuits, that have had very limited success in reversing this trend. Furthermore, it has de facto government sanction in that Medicare will cover "facility fees," and so will many private insurers (for reasons that will become apparent shortly). Every Citizen Patient should question its rationale. And while you're questioning, ask how the CEO of a private hospital system such as Novant can earn over $2 million in a year and the CEO of a "not-for-profit" hospital system such as the University of Pennsylvania's can earn over $3 million in a year. One would think they are charged with bundling subprime mortgages instead of providing a service to the ill.

UNC School of Medicine and UNC Health Care

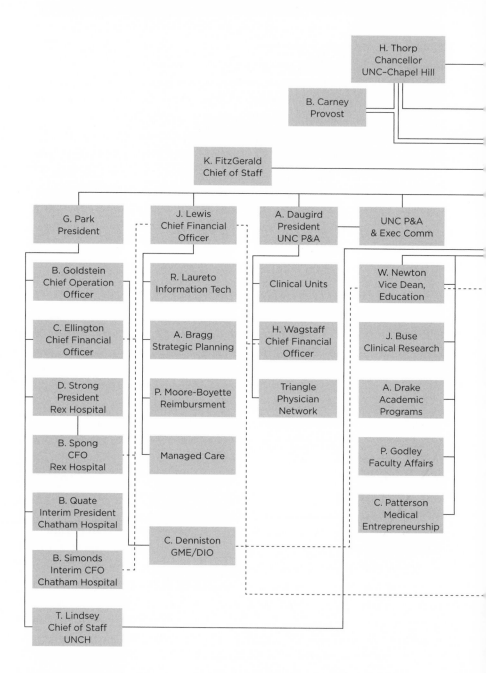

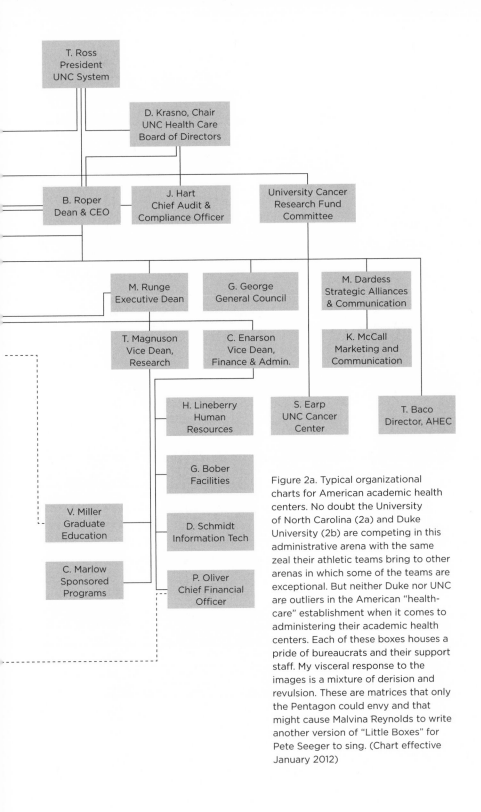

T. Ross
President
UNC System

D. Krasno, Chair
UNC Health Care
Board of Directors

B. Roper
Dean & CEO

J. Hart
Chief Audit &
Compliance Officer

University Cancer
Research Fund
Committee

M. Runge
Executive Dean

G. George
General Council

M. Dardess
Strategic Alliances
& Communication

T. Magnuson
Vice Dean,
Research

C. Enarson
Vice Dean,
Finance & Admin.

K. McCall
Marketing and
Communication

H. Lineberry
Human
Resources

S. Earp
UNC Cancer
Center

T. Baco
Director, AHEC

G. Bober
Facilities

V. Miller
Graduate
Education

D. Schmidt
Information Tech

C. Marlow
Sponsored
Programs

P. Oliver
Chief Financial
Officer

Figure 2a. Typical organizational charts for American academic health centers. No doubt the University of North Carolina (2a) and Duke University (2b) are competing in this administrative arena with the same zeal their athletic teams bring to other arenas in which some of the teams are exceptional. But neither Duke nor UNC are outliers in the American "health-care" establishment when it comes to administering their academic health centers. Each of these boxes houses a pride of bureaucrats and their support staff. My visceral response to the images is a mixture of derision and revulsion. These are matrices that only the Pentagon could envy and that might cause Malvina Reynolds to write another version of "Little Boxes" for Pete Seeger to sing. (Chart effective January 2012)

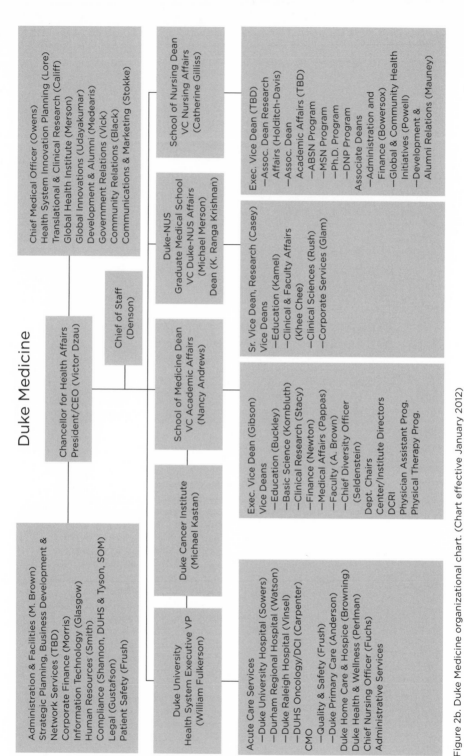

Duke Medicine

Chancellor for Health Affairs President/CEO (Victor Dzau)

Chief of Staff (Denson)

Chief Medical Officer (Owens)
Health System Innovation Planning (Lore)
Translational & Clinical Research (Califf)
Global Health Institute (Merson)
Global Innovations (Udayakumar)
Development & Alumni (Medearis)
Government Relations (Vick)
Community Relations (Black)
Communications & Marketing (Stokke)

Administration & Facilities (M. Brown)
Strategic Planning, Business Development &
Network Services (TBD)
Corporate Finance (Morris)
Information Technology (Glasgow)
Human Resources (Smith)
Compliance (Shannon, DUHS & Tyson, SOM)
Legal (Gustafson)
Patient Safety (Frush)

Duke University Health System Executive VP (William Fulkerson)

Duke Cancer Institute (Michael Kastan)

School of Medicine Dean VC Academic Affairs (Nancy Andrews)

Duke-NUS Graduate Medical School VC Duke-NUS Affairs (Michael Merson) Dean (K. Ranga Krishnan)

School of Nursing Dean VC Nursing Affairs (Catherine Gilliss)

Acute Care Services
 −Duke University Hospital (Sowers)
 −Durham Regional Hospital (Watson)
 −Duke Raleigh Hospital (Vinsel)
 −DUHS Oncology/DCI (Carpenter)
CMO
 −Quality & Safety (Frush)
 −Duke Primary Care (Anderson)
Duke Home Care & Hospice (Browning)
Duke Health & Wellness (Perlman)
Chief Nursing Officer (Fuchs)
Administrative Services

Exec. Vice Dean (Gibson)
Vice Deans
 −Education (Buckley)
 −Basic Science (Kornbluth)
 −Clinical Research (Stacy)
 −Finance (Newton)
 −Medical Affairs (Pappas)
 −Faculty (A. Brown)
 −Chief Diversity Officer
  (Seldenstein)
Dept. Chairs
Center/Institute Directors
DCRI
Physician Assistant Prog.
Physical Therapy Prog.

Sr. Vice Dean, Research (Casey)
Vice Deans
 −Education (Kamel)
 −Clinical & Faculty Affairs
  (Khee Chee)
 −Clinical Sciences (Rush)
 −Corporate Services (Glam)

Exec. Vice Dean (TBD)
 −Assoc. Dean Research
  Affairs (Holditch-Davis)
 −Assoc. Dean
  Academic Affairs (TBD)
 −ABSN Program
 −MSN Program
 −Ph.D. Program
 −DNP Program
Associate Deans
 −Administration and
  Finance (Bowersox)
 −Global & Community Health
  Initiatives (Powell)
 −Development &
  Alumni Relations (Mauney)

Figure 2b. Duke Medicine organizational chart. (Chart effective January 2012)

Most Americans under age sixty-five who have health insurance can name their insurance company: Cigna, Aetna, BCBS, etc. They are fooling themselves; rather, they are fooled by the structure of the system. The vast majority of working Americans who have health insurance are insured by their employer; the health-insurance company is merely contracted by the employer to process the claims. The business model is closer to the way the Pentagon contracts for goods and services, a "cost-plus" contract. The health-insurance company asks the employer for the money to pay for the services the employee obtained and for an additional percentage of that sum to cover the health insurer's overhead. The argument for cost-plus contracts by the Pentagon is marginal, relating to national security if a supplier goes bankrupt or cuts corners. The rationale for cost-plus contracts for health insurance is not marginal; it's perverse. It is no wonder that the health-insurance industry does not balk at facility fees or at myriad useless therapies that we will discuss in the next chapter. As the cash flowing through the coffers of the insurance companies grows, so, too, does the magnitude of their profit premium. And the larger the profit premium, the larger the financial rewards for their executives and stockholders.

MARKETING HEALTH CARE

Who do you think pays for all those full-page advertisements for hospitals, clinics, particular practices, and the latest technologies? That comes out of clinical income, too, but washed through the inventive accounting streams of the for-profit and not-for-profit hospitals and clinics. There is often a sizable staff committed to this effort. At UNC Health Care, eleven highly trained professionals currently lead the efforts of the News Office and the Department of Public Affairs and Marketing. They are hawking with the same zeal, and sometimes the same elegance, that we associate with car dealerships. But unlike automobile dealerships, which can go out of business if they sell lemons, hospital marketing is to be accepted at face value. Caveat emptor. Furthermore, this hospital-based marketing exercise coincides with the demise of the profession of health journalism. Public affairs and marketing are taking up the slack for the print and broadcast media and in cyberspace. Not only must the Citizen Patient bring a great deal of skepticism to the hospitals' advertising, but no one should let down their guard with the media. Let me explain how this works.

In the preamble to its Code of Ethics, the Society of Professional Journalism declares: "Public enlightenment is the forerunner of justice and the foundation of democracy. . . . Conscientious journalists from all media and specialties strive to serve the public with thoroughness and honesty." There were, and still are, many examples of print and broadcast journalists living up to this standard with the support of editors, producers, and publishers who knew no other way. Medical journalism is a specialty in journalism. The Association of Health Care Journalists, founded in 1997, is based at the School of Journalism of the University of Missouri and has more than 1,000 members. In its Statement of Principles, the association does not shy away from recognizing the moral hazards inherent in translating "health" news to the public:

> We should strive to be independent from the agendas and timetables of journals, advocates, and industry and government agencies. We should nourish and encourage original and analytical reporting that provides audiences/readers with context. Given that thousands of journal articles and conference presentations appear each year, and that relatively few are immediately relevant to our audiences/readers, health journalists have a responsibility to be selective so that significant news is not overwhelmed by a blizzard of trivial reports. We are the eyes and ears of our audiences/readers; we must not be mere mouthpieces for industry, government agencies, researchers or health-care providers. . . . Health care journalists should remember that their loyalties reside with the truth and with the needs of the community.

Living up to these principles is a challenge that is met unevenly. But the ethical standard is understood, and shortcomings evoke disdain in the profession.

Programs in health and medical journalism have been developed at a number of the leading schools of journalism. The program at the University of North Carolina at Chapel Hill was founded a decade ago. I have been privileged to participate on its advisory board for many years. The consensus at a recent board meeting was that health journalism is more beleaguered than most other specialties by the financial crunch that faces the entire Fourth Estate. One fallback available to editors in such a circumstance is to purchase the coverage from leading journalists in the employ of other outlets. We have grown accustomed to this when it comes to finance, politics, sports, and international coverage. This compromise applies to health reporting as well.

But health reporting has access to another source, one that is particularly appealing given its packaging and the cost. This source hides behind the euphemism "Health Communications," but in practice it resides in the various hospital public affairs and marketing departments we've just discussed. Staffing these departments are people highly skilled in communicating to the public, with backgrounds in marketing, public relations, or, increasingly, health journalism. Such jobs are all too often the soft landing for unemployed health journalists. Hence, the pronouncements and announcements are often put forth in the glossiest of multimedia formats as well as the more standard press announcements. There are websites that serve as the platform for this activity (www.futurity.org is an example).

This is not the health journalism that satisfies the ethical principles put forth by the Association of Health Care Journalists, however. We know that thanks to a study funded by the National Cancer Institute and published in the *Annals of Internal Medicine* (vol. 150 [2009]: 613–18). The academic medical centers in the study issued an average of nearly fifty press releases annually. Nearly half of them pertained to research using animals that was almost always cast as relevant to human health. Of the releases about primary human research, very few were describing studies that would pass muster as high quality; far more described findings that were preliminary at best. Most neglected to emphasize cautions regarding interpreting such studies. Clearly, academic medical centers have no compunctions about dressing up marketing in scientific garb to fool the public for selfish motives.

It is for this reason that I am so concerned about the decimation of the ranks of health journalists. I understand the appeal of "press releases" and the greater appeal of information that accumulates on websites; convenience can unburden the journalists assigned to cover more than is possible, and cost-effectiveness can unburden the publisher whose cash flow is so tenuous. However, the public is not just poorly served by this system; it is likely led astray. At the very least, media must state whether the reportage is based on primary sources that take personal responsibility for the validity of the pronouncement. Better yet, independent sources should be queried as to the validity, reproducibility, and relevance of the claims. But neither should be passed along to the public unfiltered by health journalists who are appropriately trained and willing to assume responsibility for the quality of the input. If the pronouncement is simply lifted from a marketing website, that should be disclosed. Maybe then the Citizen Patient will know to decry marketing dressed up as journalism.

Perhaps the most sophomoric of all medical marketing schemes are the many rankings: Best Doctors, Top Doctors, *U.S. News & World Report*'s many lists, and more. I have no personal bone to pick in this regard. Throughout my career, I have been listed on many of these—including the first two—often in more than one category. Truth be told, it's more fun to be listed than not; even I cannot totally suppress sophomoric ideas. These lists are useless as indicators of clinical judgment for reasons that relate to the methods used to construct them. The definition of "best" is in the eye of the beholder. It is a major methodological challenge to design questionnaires that force all respondents to look with the same rose-colored glasses. Asking one doctor to list his favored consultant is certain to evoke criteria different from that of another doctor. That's how they construct the first two lists, a mix of apples and pears. These lists are the property of private companies that are ever more inventive in the way they promote the lists, including selling "members" access to the lists and enticing the listed doctors with everything from plaques to full-page advertisements. I presume these listing companies have found a lucrative marketing niche for their unreliable, nonscientific approach to measuring "quality." That stands as witness to general gullibility and as reproach to peer review.

U.S. News & World Report is far more systematic in its approach and very successful. In fact, its lists have survived the printed magazine and anchor its legacy, a very popular website. The lists are constructed by Robert Morse and his small staff in Washington, D.C., using criteria that they have generated and honed over the years, criteria that give different weights to different attributes. Those of us who are trained to undertake definitions of "quality" know that the challenge is in defining "quality" and validating the criteria for its measurement. How do you know that what you measure is really an indicator of "quality"? When it comes to education, are you more interested in admission credentials, passing rate, or some measure of "success" down the road? For hospitals, does discharge rate reflect the selection of less-ill patients or the competence in treating more-ill patients? Is the number of publications, trainees, research grants, and so forth a valid measure, and if so, are some categories more important than others?

U.S. News & World Report has made these determinations in a fashion that is barely transparent, highly personalized, and without scientific validation. Malcolm Gladwell's "The Order of Things" (*New Yorker,*

February 14, 2011) is a brilliant critique of this process. Nonetheless, the *U.S. News & World Report* listing has become an accepted benchmark for the administration across the academic spectrum, including academic health centers. Schools such as mine have made the improvement of our ranking a high priority. After all, neighboring Duke Medical Center ranks high overall and in many categories, whereas UNC rankings are dismal by comparison. Committees are meeting. We are following the precedents set by many, many peer organizations—Weill Cornell, the University of Pittsburgh, the Mayo Clinic to mention a few that fill my mailbox with newsletters and glossy magazines. All are co-opting clinical income in this quest of recognition as if this validates "quality." All this bears witness to the shallow vision of the leadership of academic health centers, the cowed posturing of the faculty, and the flawed nature of the listings.

COMPETING FOR PATIENTS

Those running medical centers generally adhere to the same business model. The model was the brainchild of a highly remunerated consulting group. Today such consulting groups are legion and have become the handmaidens of most of the chief executives, often planting their disciples in the bureaucracy when they move on. The business model, formulated two decades ago, holds that the secret to a thriving medical center is capturing a critical number of patients in the community for the most lucrative "health-care" interventions—mainly the procedures and drug trials—performed at the center. Large hospitals compete to buy out medical practices in the community and even buy up the local hospitals that serve these practices. Medical centers incur considerable debt in this activity. There is a flaw in the business model, however. It was assumed that the physicians and hospitals would maintain the same level of fiscal productivity under contract as they did fending for themselves. That did not pan out, though, and many a medical center found itself drowning in debt. Some saw no option other than to be purchased by larger for-profit players. These include some prominent hospitals, such as the teaching hospitals at Georgetown University and the University of Louisville. Some, such as the hospital of the University of Pennsylvania, battled back from this brink.

The consulting groups and the chief executives learned a lesson, but not the lesson you might have guessed. There was nothing wrong with the business model, they decided; only its implementation needed fixing. Rather than buy out practices and hospitals, the mother hospital should build and staff explants in the community. Furthermore, not only would they build and staff primary-care facilities and general hospitals, but they would build specialty-care facilities such as imaging centers, outpatient surgery centers, their own doc-in-the-boxes, colonoscopy centers, and whatever they deemed useful to serve the business model. Of course, all this is playing out in a highly competitive marketplace. I envision the various leaders listed in Figure 2 sitting around a form of Monopoly board deciding to buy a clinic or a hospital for any particular location. The American landscape is dotted with these facilities, often with neighboring facilities owned by competing medical centers vying for the business of patients in the same neighborhood. Maybe when competing drugstore chains build stores on each corner of a large intersection, they know what they're doing. Maybe the consultants finally have their business model correct. I'm not betting on the survival of either model. They both assume that there are no Citizen Patients. They will learn.

Industry Masquerading in Academic Clothing

Very seldom anymore are the trials necessary for licensing drugs or devices (there is a crucial difference, but I'll save that for another chapter) carried out by the manufacturer. There is an industry devoted to providing that service: the Contract Research Organizations (CROs). I have long railed against this industry, as I consider it inherently conflictual. Science is the exercise of disproving any hypothesis. The CRO is contracted in the hope it will prove the hypothesis that a particular drug or device is an important enough contribution to qualify for licensing by the FDA. There is no joy at the CRO or the contracting company when the study is negative. It behooves the CRO to design the study and the data analysis in such a way as to minimize that likelihood. CROs can be very lucrative. Some employ tens of thousands of people at sites around the world. Quintiles, which pioneered the industry in the 1980s, is a privately held company with annual revenues of over $3 billion and over 20,000 employees in sixty countries. Many academic health centers have jumped on this bandwagon, creating their own CROs. Some of these, such as Duke's, are sizeable enterprises. Furthermore, many an "academic physician" is employed for "translational research," which is a euphemism for recruiting patients into trials run by CROs. CROs would have never come into existence and thrived if the pharmaceutical industry had not found outsourcing the licensing process advantageous.

To understand this, one needs an overview of the process of new drug development and of the regulation of drug licensure by the FDA. All the major pharmaceutical firms have research groups developing candidate drugs that target specific diseases. Most of this work is derivative. That means that the novel ideas are usually generated at government-supported laboratories around the resource-advantaged world, largely by virtue of government grants to basic researchers in universities or government-supported freestanding laboratories, such as the National Institutes of Health in the United States and the Medical Research Council laboratories in the United Kingdom.

There was a time when laboratories in pharmaceutical firms were a fountainhead of novel ideas and discoveries, some of the caliber that garners Nobel Prizes: Selman Waksman at the Merck Institute for streptomycin; Gertrude Elion and George Hitchings at Burroughs-Wellcome for drugs for herpes, leukemia, and gout; and John Vane, who did much of his work on the mechanisms for aspirin's effect at the Wellcome Institute. But the glory days of in-house pharmaceutical industry research are largely past. Basic research is too likely to lead to insights that have no commercial downstream. Far better to let others outside the industry make the discoveries that are promising in that regard and then pursue them in-house.

For some time, nearly all novel pharmaceuticals have had their birthing in government-supported laboratories, meaning they are fruits of the tax dollar. Somehow that gets lost in the industry's loud claims about the cost of research. The in-house research involves developing compounds that affect some biochemical pathway, which was identified elsewhere and thought to be a candidate for therapy. Once such an agent is developed, it is tested in animal models that seem to mimic human disease or some aspect of human disease. If the animals survive the treatment, their condition seems to be affected positively, and the target disease is deemed commercially important, human experimentation commences. Enter the CRO.

Some CROs specialize in the early phases of human testing and others in the later phases. For all phases, protocols have to be written and approved by an Institutional Review Board (IRB). IRBs are usually comprised of a mix of folks, including some with backgrounds in science, ethics, and law. Most IRBs are based in universities. However, some are based in hospitals and, believe it or not, in industry, including in CROs. There have been issues with the competency of IRB reviews, including in surprising quarters like Duke Medical Center, which was sanctioned by federal authorities at one point. As a result, federal oversight is considerable, although, given the number of IRBs and the number of proposals, it is hit-or-miss. When the IRB functions well, its review of a proposal is a demanding exercise emphasizing first the safety of the subjects of the study and the degree to which their consent to participate is fully informed. The degree to which the study is testing an important hypothesis—for example, that this drug works or works better than another—is a secondary issue.

The first tier of study of a new drug, Phase I, recruits normal volunteers and is designed to see if the agent is tolerated at the doses proposed. The second tier, Phase II, is similar but recruits patients. Benefiting the patients in a Phase II trial is viewed as encouraging but not necessary to go on to a Phase III trial. Both Phase I and Phase II trials are exploratory in that they recruit a limited number of subjects to answer concerns about major toxic effects. Obviously, Phase I and II trials are necessary but intrinsically scary since there may be no precedent for human exposure to the agents. They typically recruit volunteers with financial inducements, which can thwart caution if the volunteer is needy. The ethical burden on the IRB is substantial. I wish there were more emphasis on whether the potential good that might come from licensing a novel drug warrants the risk, but often the potential for good is as uncertain as the potential for harm.

Phase III trials are designed as definitive experiments carried out in patient populations. Phase III trials are the bread-and-butter of CROs and are the licensing trials for the FDA. The prototype is the double-blind randomized controlled trial (RCT). A well-defined population of patients with a particular disorder is recruited. The subjects are instructed in the details of the research protocol, including the methods, the results of the Phase I and II trials, the potential harms, and the potential benefits. They are then asked if they are willing to participate. If so, they are asked to sign a permission slip that reiterates all of this information. The entire recruitment process must have been approved by an IRB beforehand. Next, the volunteers are randomly assigned to receive either the study drug or a comparator, which is either a placebo or a licensed drug.

The protocol is termed "double-blind" when neither the investigators nor the volunteers can know if a particular individual received the study drug or the comparator. Dosing and the details of monitoring the subjects for benefit and for harm are also detailed in the protocol that was approved by the IRB. There may be independent investigators who have access to the data as it unfolds in case there is a dramatic effect—harm in particular—in which case, the study is aborted. But otherwise, the protocol's constraints on dosing, duration, and outcome measures must be adhered to if the results are to be interpretable. The hypothesis is that there is no difference between the effects of the study drug and those of the comparator. The design calls for statistical tests trying to reject that hypothesis. Everyone is pleased if the hypothesis is rejected because the study drug proved beneficial with little if any harm. It is all so elegant—but there are many devils in the details that need to be flushed into broad daylight so that no Citizen Patient is ever bamboozled by "evidence" again. Here, we'll look at some of the bamboozling that relates to the process of licensing drugs. In the next chapter, we'll take on the bamboozling that relates to making an informed medical decision.

MASSAGING DATA

Phase III trials have become enormous undertakings, often recruiting many thousands of subjects and generating contracts for CROs worth many millions of dollars. Why? If one is studying a disease that kills nearly everyone within a year of diagnosis, such as metastatic lung or pancreatic cancer, shouldn't it be easy to find out if the study drug is a cure? You could recruit twenty patients, give half of them the drug, and wait to see whether all on the drug were disease free a year later and all on the placebo were dead. If you had such a drug, the independent scientists monitoring the trial would likely spot this difference early and abort the trial so that all on the placebo were switched to the study drug. In fact, one might have even detected this hallelujah drug in its Phase II trial. But hallelujah drugs for horrible diseases come along so very, very infrequently that drug development on that basis would be fatuous.

Hence all Phase III trials are designed to detect something less than hallelujah. Let's say one would settle for saving one life in twenty patients, which all of us would consider a worthwhile effort if we weren't causing too much harm to those not saved. Obviously, a trial with only ten patients on the study drug has only a 50 percent chance of saving one life. Even if the difference in survival between the patients on the study group and the placebo group is one in ten, that could easily happen by chance. This is a lethal disease that "kills nearly everyone within a year of diagnosis," but not everyone. Some live a little longer treated or not, and the occasional "outlier" patient lives longer yet. You would need to recruit more patients into the study to detect saving the life of one in twenty patients, but not a great many more. It would require numbers in the hundreds for the study to have the "statistical power" to detect this difference. A Phase III RCT with a couple hundred subjects that lasts a year to detect a dramatic benefit in one out of twenty patients is not burdensome in terms of cost, recruitment, or investigator time. It's also not as demanding in data analysis. But . . .

The drug development enterprise has grown so large and greedy that it can't be sustained by the occasional highly effective, quasi-hallelujah new product. It is wedded to licensing drugs that are far less effective, both in terms of the likelihood they will advantage any patient and the degree to which that patient is advantaged. For example, there are drugs licensed for the treatment of metastatic lung and prostate cancer on the basis of a statistical argument that they prolong life a matter of months. Then there are all the drugs licensed for effects on outcomes that are not as unequivocal as death (or heart attacks, or kidney failure, or the like). These are the drugs that ameliorate symptoms such as pain, sadness, heartburn, etc. Quantifying these "soft" outcomes is very challenging; a patient can easily end up with a bit less insomnia but more fatigue, for example. Nonetheless, the pharmaceutical industry would rather market marginal drugs to a large population than hope to develop a truly effective drug for a small market.

Furthermore, they are in a hurry to get these marginal drugs to market to satisfy their profit motives and those of their stockholders. Trials with thousands of subjects are the rule, as are outcome measures that are soft if not surrogate and composite. A surrogate outcome measures something that relates to disease but not disease itself; cholesterol is a good example. A composite outcome is a cluster of hard and soft, such as fatal and nonfatal heart attacks + heart failure + heart pain (angina) + need for heart surgery; it takes a canny reader of these results to realize how often only the last measure is all that changed and that a "need for surgery" is in the eyes of the surgeon rather than a reliable clinical outcome measure.

Running these enormous trials and mining the even more enormous data sets they generate is a considerable undertaking that is generally outsourced to CROS. These trials are too large to carry out in a single research site; they are multisite and require escalating organizational skills. Never do these trials proceed without hitches: results are incomplete, patients drop out or cross over to alternative therapies, study sites differ in adherence to protocols, and much more. There is always a need to apply critical eyes to the data in the course of its analysis. That's when the conflictual nature of the CRO industry comes into play. When a scientist is faced with this morass in the academy, the pressure is to err on the side of conservatism—that is, to assume in the analysis that any inadequacy in the data prejudices against a positive result. Subliminally, the CRO operates under a different pressure. Sometimes, it's not so subliminal: criminal charges have been brought against several individuals working with or for CROs. The issue is sufficiently critical that there is federal oversight, even when the CRO is offshore. Nonetheless, as we've already discussed, studies managed by CROs are far more likely to prove positive than studies on the same drug sponsored by governments.

RECRUITING SUBJECTS

Some twenty-five years ago, I made the tongue-in-cheek comment that most trials for rheumatoid arthritis were carried out in the same 300 patients. That's because there were rheumatologists who were handmaidens of the pharmaceutical industry and who had a "stable" of patients they paid to volunteer for study after study. There still are such physicians, in all specialties, who have their stable of patients but now are handmaidens for CROs. In fact, their numbers are growing, as is the size of their stables, in large part because these "drug trialists" are handsomely compensated for their efforts. The subject-patients may or may not be compensated, but their medical/surgical care is only compensated to the degree stipulated by the RCT protocol. All other care, including care relating to the disease being treated in the study, is covered by whatever insurance mechanism is available to them. So the drug trialists are paid for monitoring the subject-patient's progress in the trial and paid again for whatever other services they provide the subject-patient. Many of the drug trialists have diamonds on their pinkies or in their ears for all this effort.

But we're talking about many trials for many diseases that need to recruit thousands of subjects. The demand is outstripping both the number of trialists and the subject pool. There are companies that contract to the CROs for the purpose of recruiting subjects. But even this is not sufficient. All of these gargantuan trials are multisite, but no longer are they multisite just in the resource-advantaged world. CROs are popping up all over, from sub-Saharan Africa to South Asia and Southeast Asia. Needless to say, oversight of trials is rapidly becoming as gargantuan a task as the performance of trials. One is wise to feel uncertain about the quality of the data that are massaged to look for the small effects. Given the cultural differences in experiencing and expressing symptoms, I'm not even certain such trials can ever discern meaningful small differences in "soft" outcomes. Bamboozling is getting ever more inventive and expensive.

SEED TRIALS

And I mean inventive. The pharmaceutical industry puts enormous effort into hiring "detail" people, a sales force to "educate" physicians on the reasons they should find the drug samples they provide as particularly indicated for the treatment of patients. It has long been known that once physicians get comfortable with a drug, meaning familiar with the dosing and the side effects, they will prescribe the drug for some time to come. That's the reason pharmaceutical marketing targets the trainees of teaching hospitals and the committees of hospitals responsible for the formulary (list of available drugs) whenever permitted.

There's another trick to serve this agenda: the "seed trial." Many of the RCTs are not testing the effectiveness of novel agents; they are looking at subtle indications for drug usage of licensed drugs or are comparing licensed drugs that are relatively similar if one examines the data from their licensing RCTs. The pharmaceutical industry might claim that they are pushing back the frontiers of ignorance with these efforts. It just happens that they are also recruiting as drug trialists doctors who were not familiar with their drug and who have influence in their communities, so-called thought leaders. These are called seed trials. They are folding the marketing budget into the research budget. Pharmaceutical firms like to hide their enormous marketing expenditures in this fashion. Like seed trials, much of sponsored educational activity serves a marketing agenda. I'm offended and saddened that so many physicians can be bought in this fashion. Citizen Patients should be also. Furthermore, no patient should agree to participate in any drug trial without assurance that the intent of the trial is meaningful—that it is designed to learn if there is a meaningful benefit for patients and not just stakeholders.

OFF-LABEL AND COMPASSIONATE USE

Drugs are licensed based on RCTs carried out on particular patient populations for particular indications. However, once a drug is licensed, there is no formal constraint on prescribing it. Physicians can decide to prescribe a drug that was licensed for treatment of one disease for the treatment of another. This is called "off-label" use because the drug is licensed only for particular indications that are noted in its labeling. This doesn't happen willy-nilly very often. For example, a new drug licensed for the treatment of patients who have retained fluid because of heart failure might be tried on a patient with liver failure who has also retained fluid. If the tried-and-true drugs have not proved effective in the patient with liver failure, it might seem perfectly reasonable to try the new fluid pill. Of course, the patient might not respond to the new drug either, or he might get worse, and there's no way to know from this empirical event whether the drug harmed his liver so as to exacerbate the fluid retention.

Off-label use is often tempered by peer interactions, but in this era of aggressive care, the outcome of peer review is more likely "Why not?" than "What if?" Part of aggressiveness at the bedside is the assumption that therapeutic cleverness is more likely to render the doctor a hero than to lead to malpractice suits. If the patient fares poorly, the assumption is that the disease would not yield even to therapeutic cleverness. Off-label use is a slippery slope. To be fair, the slope is greased by some legendary observations when treatment for one indication did something good for a coincident disease. That's how we learned that Viagra did little for heart pain but much for erectile dysfunction. But it's a slippery slope for the well-being of the patient. I am viscerally disinclined to prescribe off-label. The only exceptions might be instances when the licensed drug is ineffective or poorly tolerated and there is a very similar drug on the formulary that has not been studied in this setting. Then I might yield, but only after a detailed discussion of the rationale with my patient and my colleagues. However, some specialties, such as oncology, are well known for having little compunction when it comes to off-label prescribing.

There is a more subtle aspect to off-label prescribing. Most licensing RCTs restrict the patient population by disease severity, age, coincidental disease, and the like. Once a drug is licensed, it is common practice and sensible to treat for the licensed indication in patients who do not quite fit the criteria used to recruit subjects for the RCT. It is possible that treating the same disease in an older patient, or in one with another coincident disease like kidney failure, will have a different outcome than would be predicted from the RCT. Today, there is no systematic way for us to know this except by the uneven operation of peer education and the even-more-uneven mechanism of reporting adverse events to the FDA. There is a serious attempt to develop a systematic way to accomplish post-licensing surveillance for unexpected good and adverse events. Such an undertaking has been called a Phase IV trial, and the Veterans Administration is developing the methodology for their patients. This is an effort that is long overdue.

The extreme of off-label use is "compassionate use." Phase I, II, and III drug trials are driven by the escalating belief on the part of investigators and pharmaceutical firms that the drug will really work; otherwise, why undertake the trials? Such a belief has a tendency to permeate the settings where trials are undertaken and the stock market where good results are anticipated. Some of these drugs are under study for the treatment of desperately ill patients. The belief that a study drug really works can often be found at the bedside of the desperately ill patient, often deposited there by caring family and caregivers. Furthermore, the handmaiden to this belief is that circumstances are too desperate to wait for the results of the RCT, let alone for licensure, before treating the patient.

The banner of "What do we have to lose?" is hoisted aloft, and the pharmaceutical firm is petitioned for release of the drug for compassionate use in this desperately ill patient. Resistance from the firm can be met with very public, sometimes litigious accusations of callous disregard for the life of a loved one. This heated battle often torments the suffering participants and elicits empathy from all who witness the anguish. That's why we need a far more dispassionate discussion in the abstract, a discussion that informs the patient and the patient's community before any such battle is joined. The truth is that most study drugs for desperate situations prove ineffective or minimally effective when all is said and done. A hallelujah drug is a rare discovery, much rarer than a drug that turns out to be harmful.

Compassionate use is a far more slippery slope than off-label use. This, in small part, is because the toxic potential of licensed drugs has been determined at least in the patients who participated in the licensing trials. Compassionate use may not be compassionate for the desperately ill loved one or anyone else, and we won't know that unless licensing trials are allowed to mature. The issue is not simply academic or scientific—it's ethical. Without demanding a demonstration of a reasonable benefit-to-risk ratio, we will do all sorts of harm and be none the wiser.

There is a counterargument. What if the drug looks really promising in the Phase II trial? Shouldn't we do away with the requirement for a Phase III trial and just license such a drug? In an ideal world, that would be a compelling argument for a real hallelujah drug. But this is not an ideal world in general and for drug trials in particular. Patients are not recruited into Phase II trials without prejudice. One is looking for patients who can tolerate the protocol and are not too sick to respond in real time. In other words, Phase II trials are designed for a purpose other than efficacy; they are designed to discern toxicity. Because of randomization, the status of the patient in a Phase III trial is less critical, as is the presence of confounders like coincidental disease. I argue vigorously for Phase III trials for the licensure of any drug in any setting. If you think it's a hallelujah drug, the trial need not be lengthy and the study population need not be large. But randomization and adherence to protocol must not be corrupted.

Direct-to-Consumer Advertising of Prescription Drugs

Until the 1980s, direct-to-consumer (DTC) advertising of prescription drugs was unheard of. It made little sense to advertise a commodity that the consumers were not allowed to purchase by their own volition. It took a peculiar intellect to realize that the consumer might be encouraged to persuade the prescriber, or that DTC advertising would capture prescribers' interest directly. In the 1980s, the testing of the DTC waters was sporadic. In the United States, it met with stringent and onerous requirements from the FDA, which limited DTC advertising to price comparisons and little else.

New Zealand sanctioned DTC advertising of prescription drugs in 1981. No other country has followed suit, with the exception of the United States. In the United States, the argument for a similarly liberal sanction has always been the protection of freedom of information and of speech. But how could one assure that the content of DTC advertising primarily served this platform and not the profit structure of the purveyors? In 1997 the FDA came out with guidelines that were not that onerous; the content of the advertising could not overstate the basis for licensure or understate concerns about toxicity. In other words, there could be no claim for benefit beyond that encompassed by licensure, and there must be some adequate presentation of potential harms. Today, U.S. broadcast media spew DTC advertisements for all sorts of pharmaceuticals, with professional actors pitching dramatically over a sotto voce litany of potential adverse effects.

This is not to say that DTC advertising has supplanted other marketing programs; to the contrary (see Figure 1). However, it is estimated that the total annual advertising expenditures for the entire pharmaceutical industry surpassed the $30 billion mark in 2005 and continue apace. It is the hand that feeds much of commercial television and the print media. And, as we discussed above, few in power in the media are willing to bite that hand.

Neither is the pharmaceutical industry lacking in zeal for DTC marketing (Figure 1). There is plenty of evidence that DTC marketing increases sales (Julie M. Donohue and others, "A Decade of Direct-to-Consumer Advertising of Prescription Drugs," *New England Journal of Medicine* 357 [2007]: 673–81). There is also a growing appreciation of the degree to which DTC advertising of prescription drugs is finding a home with interactive Internet media (Brian Liang and Timothy Mackey, "Direct-to-Consumer Advertising with Interactive Internet Medias: Global Regulation and Public Health Issues," *Journal of the American Medical Association* 305 [2011]: 824–25). This trend raises fascinating issues in terms of global regulation and public health. No doubt these issues will have to be addressed, but there is every reason to wonder whether they can be addressed effectively by regulatory means. We will do much better if the world is populated with enlightened Citizen Patients.

The Hidden Agendas of the Disease Societies

Nearly every disease known to man has an advocacy group, a not-for-profit organization chartered to promote care and support research to benefit those who suffer from the particular disease. Today, these are separated from the professional societies that advocate for practitioners of particular clinical specialties like the American Colleges of Medicine, Cardiology, Rheumatology, etc. Most of the disease foundations were started by well-meaning, prominent physicians interested in particular diseases suffered by their patients. All are now lay organizations, often with advisory boards and usually leadership from the relevant professionals. They are meant to be philanthropies rather than medical guilds. In fact, to maintain their special tax-free status, the disease foundations were forced to separate from the professional organizations that specialize in the care of patients with the same disease.

The primordial American Heart Association (AHA) was originally the Association for the Prevention and Relief of Heart Disease, founded in New York City in 1915 by physicians and social workers. Similar groups formed in other cities and coalesced into the AHA in 1924. In 1948, to broaden the organization's scope of activities, people from many walks of life were brought into the fold, and fund-raising went public. By 1975 the AHA had many chapters, raised funds on a national scale, and supported educational programs and research. That was the year I was awarded an Established Investigatorship from the AHA, which paid my salary for five years while I was an assistant professor at UNC and freed me up to do laboratory science.

This was also about the time when cardiology was transforming from the realm of the exquisitely competent bedside clinician to entrepreneurship in terms of both interventional cardiology and cardiovascular pharmaceuticals. Enormous support has flowed from the manufacturers of the relevant widgets and pills. Symbiotically, the AHA has been an advocate for the use of both the widgets and the drugs. The AHA's medical leadership and "educational agenda" are front and center in "helping" America understand the virtues of the sponsors' products without discussing the possibility that the products are not helpful. The AHA is now an enormous enterprise that walks a fine line between patient advocacy and marketing for its stakeholders.

The Arthritis Foundation (AF) was organized in 1948 as the Arthritis and Rheumatism Foundation and soon merged with the professional organization, the American Rheumatism Association (ARA), which dominated in the early years. The ARA transformed into the American College of Rheumatology (ACR) in 1986 and split off from the AF. The early AF was indeed philanthropic; the input of the ARA was beyond reproach. In fact, the early leaders of the ARA were the pioneers of American rheumatology, including some of my mentors. No one made money, directly or indirectly. Today, both the AF and the ACR are dripping in conflicts of interest. AF publications are riddled with advertising, and the organization is fat with corporate sponsorship. The ACR is worse on both accounts.

All of this is following the precedent of the American Cancer Society (ACS). The ACS began as the American Society for the Control of Cancer (ASCC) in 1913, founded by prominent physicians and incorporated a decade later by prominent businessmen. After World War II, the ASCC was reorganized as the ACS and a fund-raising campaign was initiated, spearheaded by the educational agenda, "Cancer's Danger Signals." Many public-relations and funding campaigns followed, including the lobbying that led to the "War on Cancer" in the Nixon administration. These were the years that saw the National Institutes of Health (NIH) evolve from a handful of institutes to a gaggle as a reflection of the growing influence of the disease-specific advocacy groups, each lobbying Congress for a distinctive presence in the NIH. The National Cancer Institute gained in every way. By 1990 the ACS had enormous wealth in liquid and nonliquid assets. In 1991 it raised $350 million, mainly from small donors. In 1992 the

American Cancer Foundation was founded, allowing for sizeable contributions and headed by a board that included executives from Amgen and Lederle, companies with much invested in cancer treatments. By 1998 the ACS had a war chest of $1 billion and an annual budget of $350 million. It was an organization with clout in Washington, D.C., and in the world of oncology outside the Beltway. Today, there are 3,400 local offices and some 2 million volunteers carrying on the mission. However, the story of the ACS is stained by well-documented episodes of misdirected goals and greed.

Economists James T. Bennett of George Washington University and Thomas J. DiLorenzo of Loyola University in Baltimore and a professor of Occupational and Environmental Medicine at the University of Illinois's School of Public Health, Samuel S. Epstein, M.D., have published extensively, accusing the ACS of abuses of its public responsibilities. All three have their own agendas, but some of their muckraking struck home. In the mid-1990s, the ACS was brought to task because of the enormous "overhead" of some of its chapters and its even more enormous accumulated wealth, which included real estate holdings. Today, the ACS is not so different from similar organizations, although the seven-figure salaries of some of its executives still raise eyebrows. But less discussed are the interlocking relationships with industry, the lobbying budget, organizational salaries and assets, and the cost and cost-effectiveness of the "educational" agenda.

Since we all are inclined to do our best to support the disease charity of our choice, it behooves the Citizen Patient to demand much more transparency in the operations of all of them.

The Crestor Canard

It's time to cement all of these provisos and forewarnings with a concrete example. They are easy to find. We'll use the recent marketing of Crestor, a statin-class drug designed to lower cholesterol. AstraZeneca is not known for passive marketing of its products. Its attempt to position Crestor ahead of the competition in this "blockbuster" market, however, pushed the limits even for the FDA, which forced AstraZeneca to pull back in its claims (Gardiner Harris, "F.D.A. Calls Ads for Cholesterol Pill Crestor 'False and Misleading,'" *New York Times*, December 23, 2004). The company still managed to spend nearly $170 million in 2007 on DTC advertising, outspending the competition and outpacing their sales. Next, AstraZeneca set out to find a reason to take Crestor beyond the indication for which it was licensed, the treatment of the surrogate measure "high cho-lesterol." Perhaps Crestor could offer something of value to individuals whose cholesterol was not defined as "high." That would be a bonanza.

On March 31, 2008, AstraZeneca trumpeted the early closing of the JUPITER trial in company announcements. The results after only two years yielded "unequivocal evidence" that their cholesterol-lowering statin, Crestor, was too effective to withhold it from anyone who was well and had normal cholesterol levels but had an elevation in another normal blood constituent, the C-reactive protein (CRP). As we will discuss in the next chapter, I am the skeptical physician who is unwilling to let anyone test my cholesterol until I see unequivocal data that taking a statin yields meaningful benefit for me. Now AstraZeneca wants me to get my CRP measured so that I can swallow Crestor if it's elevated. On November 9, 2008, the results of JUPITER were finally published in the *New England Journal Medicine*. I knew at the time that there was a devil in the details. Let me flush it out for you.

AstraZeneca invested a great deal in this Herculean drug trial. They contracted with physicians in over 1,300 centers in twenty-six countries to recruit subjects. Some 90,000 were screened, and nearly 18,000 en-rolled. At each center, half the recruits were randomly assigned to swal-low a placebo pill and the other half Crestor. The intent was to monitor this army of volunteers for five years to see if the groups differed in their incidence of a composite outcome comprised of any of the following: heart attack, stroke, hospitalization for unstable angina or for surgery on their coronary arteries, and death from cardiovascular causes. JUPITER, as is true for all modern trials, had an oversight committee charged with breaking the code periodically to see if the volunteers on Crestor were faring better or worse than the volunteers on placebo. The JUPITER over-sight committee was comprised of luminaries in the world of cardiology who, like nearly all the principal JUPITER trial investigators, had declared financial involvements with the industry that serves the cardiovascular enterprise, many with AstraZeneca. After 1.9 years, the oversight commit-tee sounded the alarm when they noted a highly statistically significant reduction in the incidence of these feared outcomes, a reduction of 56 percent. The trial was terminated; AstraZeneca trumpeted the benefit of Crestor and stockholders took notice.

A reduction of 56 percent is hard to ignore—at first blush—but the real numbers behind that tell a much less dramatic story. At the end of two years, about 2 percent of the volunteers suffered one of the cardio-vascular events in the composite. For the Crestor group, 1.6 percent suffered such an event, whereas 2.8 percent of those not afforded Crestor did so—a difference of 1.2 percent. Not all of these people were in the trial all of the first two years, however; they entered at different times, reflecting the vagaries of recruitment. A more accurate measurement that takes this into account is to calculate for every 100 people how many would have suffered one of the cardiovascular outcomes in a year in the trial. This event rate for any of the events is 0.77 for those on Crestor and 1.36 among those who did not receive the drug. That's the 56 percent reduction that is being trumpeted. That means I'd have to treat about 200 well people with Crestor for a year to spare one of these cardiovascular events. And if you parse the composite outcome, the result is even less impressive: I'd have to treat about 400 well people for a year to spare 1 a heart attack and about 600 to spare 1 a stroke. I am unwilling even to suggest a life-saving benefit.

So the reduction of 56 percent may be hard to ignore, but it calls for careful consideration rather than prescribing zeal. Yet this reduction in a very small outcome to an even smaller outcome fueled an enormous DTC advertising campaign, was detailed to countless physicians, and was emphasized in countless continuing medical-education events. Consider the following three questions.

Should the trial have been stopped early? The monitoring committee's major responsibility is to the safety of the volunteers. If there was a hint of untoward toxicity, stopping prematurely was justified. One might argue that if a substantial benefit was apparent early on, stopping the trial and switching the volunteers who were on placebo to the active drug would be ethical. But stopping for small differences in the direction of benefit is not justifiable. Small differences come and go almost randomly during the course of these prolonged, enormous trials. Sitting there with bated breath and waiting for a positive wobble is an unjustifiable act of cherry-picking. I wonder if the oversight committee, given all their conflictual relationships, considered this.

Are you convinced that this small effect is real, that it will reproduce if one were to repeat the JUPITER trial? I am not, as a corollary to my answer to the first rhetorical question. I am reflexively skeptical of effects of this magnitude. My main reason relates to the nature of the randomized controlled trials. There are many factors vying to seal a well person's cardiovascular fate. For example, there are the so-called cardiovascular risk factors, such as obesity and tobacco abuse. By assigning volunteers randomly to Crestor or placebo, one hopes that the number of smokers and obese folks are equal in the two groups. When the JUPITER investigators checked, indeed such measurable risk factors were distributed 50:50.

One has to have faith that the factors that cannot be safely measured (such as the degree to which the blood vessels are diseased) also distribute 50:50. This could be measured if all these well volunteers were subjected to coronary angiography, but that would be unethical; cardiac catheterization is a miserable experience that bumps off a percent or two—hardly a tolerable price to pay to measure the degree of coronary artery disease in the volunteers.

Other important confounding variables could have been ethically measured, but JUPITER was designed to ignore them, assuming they distributed 50:50 between the Crestor-exposed and placebo-exposed subjects; socioeconomic status, job security, and education level are important risk factors that are independent of those measured and likely to vary widely across the research sites in these twenty-six countries. Slight imbalances between the Crestor and placebo groups in the unmeasured and immeasurable confounders could result in effects of the magnitude touted by JUPITER. I never leap to act on the basis of such small effects. It's why this year if you feed your family margarine, you're not a caring person, while not long ago, it was butter that was bad for you.

If you're convinced these small effects are real, are they meaningful to you? Are you willing to swallow Crestor every day for two years in the hopes you're the one in hundreds who just might be spared a nonfatal heart attack? Does it bother you that more of the volunteers on Crestor were diagnosed with diabetes? Aside from diabetes, the volunteers for JUPITER were not harmed in the two years. But that does not mean the drug is risk free. Does it bother you that the occasional person on Crestor dies from muscle disease caused by Crestor, and some have liver or kidney irritation? I am not tormented by such uncertainties, as I doubt the small effects are real and therefore have no interest in taking or prescribing Crestor. You and your prescribing physician should take pause at the very least. The Citizen Patient is outraged.

However, the JUPITER investigators and AstraZeneca do not share my compunctions. Rather, they take refuge in several of the tenets of contemporary small-effect epidemiology. They believe that these small effects are real. Furthermore, they believe that the small effects recognized in the first two years are likely to prove cumulative and therefore grow as the years pass. It's this belief that triggered the halting of the trial. And finally, they believe that the small likelihood of a good effect for an individual translates into a major public-health benefit; benefiting one in a hundred means benefiting 1,000 in every million. Obviously, AstraZeneca has a vested interest in holding on to these beliefs as firmly as possible. So does the lead author and investigator on JUPITER, Paul Ridker, who holds a patent on the measurement of the form of CRP that triggers treatment. He holds this patent in conjunction with his home institution, Harvard's Brigham Hospital, whose CRO was contracted to carry out JUPITER. To make matters even worse, Ridker's argument that his measurement of CRP is measuring anything meaningful is untenable. The Citizen Patient will not be surprised to learn that the JUPITER trial is not reproducible. The Heart Protection Study Collaborative Group analyzed the data for the 20,000 patients in their statin RCT to demonstrate that CRP is irrelevant ("C-Reactive Protein Concentration and the Vascular Benefits of Statin Therapy: An Analysis of 20,536 Patients in the Heart Protection Study," *Lancet* 377 [2011]: 469–76).

2

Price Fixing

Americans support an enormous enterprise in the American health-care system. To do so, we expend nearly 20 percent of the gross domestic product of this country. No other citizenry commits half as much to their health-care system. What are we purchasing with this largesse? Why are we outstripping all sister nations, many of which have enviable health outcomes compared to ours? This chapter is a primer on how we set those prices.

Birthing the Beast

The Agency for Healthcare Research and Quality (AHRQ), tucked into the Department of Health and Human Services, is charged with an array of missions from monitoring health-care parameters to funding research aimed at improving outcomes. As part of the former, AHRQ maintains a Medical Expenditure Panel Survey (MEPS) collecting data as to how many civilian adults are treated, what they are treated for, and at what expense. This is a challenging undertaking since the only readily available data relate to Medicare recipients. All other data sets are fragmented and often difficult to monitor reliably. There are also challenges to the validity of the disease categories, the reliability of cost estimates, and the handling of the data on individuals with multiple diseases. Data collection and analysis take a lot of time, effort, and compromise. Nonethe-

TABLE 1. Total Expenditures on the Ten Most Costly Conditions among Adults Age Eighteen and Older in 2008 (in Billions of Dollars)

CATEGORY	WOMEN	MEN
Heart disease	43.6	47.3
Cancer	37.7	33.7
Mental disorders	37.3	22.6
Trauma-related disorders	34.1	33.2
Osteoarthritis	33.2	23.0
Pulmonary diseases	26.8	17.7
Hypertension	25.9	21.4
Diabetes	23.2	22.3
Back problems	20.2	14.4
Lipid abnormalities	18.0	20.5

Source: Center for Financing, Access, and Cost Trends, Agency for Healthcare Research and Quality, Household Component of Medical Expenditure Panel Survey (2008).

less, MEPS offers the best window on health expenditures in the United States. The overview for 2008 was published in July 2011 as Statistical Brief #331 (http://www.meps.ahrq.gov/mepsweb/data_files/publications/st331/stat331.shtml).

In 2008 the cost of treating patients for heart disease topped $47 billion for men and $44 billion for women, leading all categories, but not by much. Cancer was the second-most-costly disease to treat at $34 billion for men and $38 billion for women. Other categories are fuzzier but nearly as impressive in expenditures (Table 1). For heart disease, trauma-related disorders, osteoarthritis, and back problems, the cost per patient is skewed by very costly surgical and imaging procedures, such as coronary artery stents, joint replacements, and spinal fusions. This is most impressive for the "Heart Disease" category: the treatment of heart disease transfers as much wealth as treatment of diseases in the "Cancer" category while treating only a third as many patients (Table 2). In some of the categories, nearly all of the wealth is transferred directly to the pharmaceutical industry and its fellow travelers.

That's true for the "Hypertension," "Diabetes," and "Lipid Abnormalities" categories—over $131 billion transferred into those coffers in 2008. And the source of the money stream is split largely and nearly equally between the employer and the taxpayer for the three most costly categories. The "Other" category in Table 3 has a considerable contribution

TABLE 2. Number of Adults and Expenditure per Adult Reporting the Ten Most Costly Conditions in 2008

CATEGORY	WOMEN	MEN
Heart disease	11.7 million–$3,723/person	10.8 million–$4,363/person
Cancer	8.4 million–$4,484/person	6.9 million–$4,873/person
Mental disorders	21.4 million–$1,739/person	11.4 million–$1,975/person
Trauma-related disorders	13.8 million–$2,475/person	12.6 million–$2,635/person
Osteoarthritis	21.4 million–$1,548/person	13.2 million–$1,749/person
Pulmonary diseases	21.5 million–$1,245/person	13.3 million–$1,324/person
Hypertension	29.5 million–$879/person	25.6 million–$838/person
Diabetes	10.9 million–$2,127/person	10.0 million–$2,219/person
Back problems	9.9 million–$2,034/person	7.5 million–$1,192/person
Lipid abnormalities	22.3 million–$810/person	22.0 million–$933/person

Source: Center for Financing, Access, and Cost Trends, Agency for Healthcare Research and Quality, Household Component of Medical Expenditure Panel Survey (2008).

TABLE 3. Distribution of Total Expenditures for Men/Women by Source of Payment in 2008 (All Figures Percentages)

SOURCE OF PAYMENT	TRAUMA	CANCER	HEART DISEASE
Private	46.3/42.3	46.0/48.5	41.2/27.8
Out-of-pocket	7.3/8.2	6.1/7.2	6.0/5.6
Medicare	20.2/32.2	32.8/30.7	38.1/52.0
Medicaid	3.0/6.7	6.6/7.1	6.1/8.8
Other	23.1/10.6	8.5/6.5	8.6/5.8

Source: Center for Financing, Access, and Cost Trends, Agency for Healthcare Research and Quality, Household Component of Medical Expenditure Panel Survey (2008).

from government-sponsored programs for various categories of retirees. The "Private" category is a euphemism, since nearly all who have "private" health insurance are provided such as a benefit of their employment, although more and more employees are asked to share in this cost by virtue of deductibles and co-pays. Furthermore, the employer contribution reduces the employers' corporate tax burden, thereby further passing costs on to taxpayers.

In my earlier books, and in several chapters of this book, I approached

TABLE 4. Health Expenditures per Capita in 2007 [a]

RANGE	COUNTRIES
>$6,000 (U.S.)	United States
$5,000–6,000	None
$4,000–5,000	Switzerland, Luxembourg, Norway
$3,000–4,000	Iceland, Australia, Netherlands, Austria, Belgium, Canada, France, Germany
$2,000–3,000	Ireland, Finland, Spain, New Zealand, Sweden, Japan, Denmark, United Kingdom, Italy, Greece
<$2,000	Israel, Singapore, Slovenia, Portugal, Korea, Cyprus

[a]This is the sum of public and private expenditure (in purchasing-power parity terms in U.S. dollars) divided by the population. Health expenditure includes the provision of health services (preventive and curative), family-planning activities, nutrition activities, and emergency aid designated for health, but it excludes the provision of water and sanitation.

Source: United Nations Human Development Report (2007) (hdr.undp.org).

the "health-care dollar" from the perspective of efficacy. In chapter 3, we will examine the efficacy, or rather the lack of efficacy, of high-ticket items such as elective orthopedics and interventional cardiology and cardio-vascular surgery for coronary artery disease. If we take just these categories into account, nearly half of the direct cost of the "health-care" purchases are useless or nearly useless interventions. Here, I want to examine how interventions are priced, useful or not.

Let's start with a little transnational perspective. At about the time the data we've just examined (Tables 1–3) were compiled, the United States was expending over $6,000 per person annually for "health care." No other country in the resource-advantaged world comes close to that figure (Table 3). But we are buying very little bang for all these extra bucks. The Commonwealth Fund published a particularly telling analysis in September 2011 (http://www.commonwealthfund.org/Publi cations/In-the-Literature/2011/Sep/Variations-in-Amenable-Mortality .aspx). They used World Health Organization mortality files and Centers for Disease Control (CDC) mortality files for the United States to determine age-standardized death rates before age seventy-five in 2006–2007 across many of the countries listed in Table 4. The notion is that the prevention of death before one's time should be most amenable to modern medical care. In the United States, nearly 1 out of every 1,000 people under age seventy-five succumbed, usually to heart disease and the like.

Citizens in no country in this study beat the United States through the Pearly Gates. In many countries, including France, Australia, Italy, Japan, Norway, Sweden, and Holland, this death rate is almost halved. In fact, by almost any measure of health and well-being, the United States lags behind all or nearly all of the countries in Table 4 to a substantial degree. Anyone who thinks the United States should preserve its health-care delivery system as it is because it's the "best" is deluded.

Who sets the fee structure in the United States? The answer is the result of fifty years of twists and turns. In *Rethinking Aging*, I discussed the politics that resulted in the legislation for Medicare in the Johnson administration. Leading the opposition was much of the medical profession, with the American Medical Association (AMA) in the vanguard. Fifty years ago, the AMA was a potent monolith that aggressively promoted the exclusive right of physicians to minister to the ill and to have independence in doing so for whatever fee the trade would bear. The notion of federal underwriting smacked of "socialized medicine," a neologism that borrowed from the national fear of the "Red" threat to the American way of life. Ayn Rand in literature and Friedrich Hayek in economics were beacons. The fact that so many elderly Americans faced their last years destitute and without access to medical care was the price of clinical autonomy and of maintaining a free market.

President Johnson and his associates were not persuaded, however, and they proposed a compromise. In exchange for federal indemnification of medical care for the elderly, the medical profession would have the right to receive "usual and customary" fees for services deemed appropriate by treating physicians. Pricing for the care of the elderly was no longer simply what the trade would bear; pricing was to be negotiated as a political process targeting the federal administration of Medicare. On July 30, 1965, the United States got Medicare, a national health-insurance scheme for our elderly citizens—albeit over half a century after nearly all of Europe had universal health care. The "usual and customary" compromise was the ticking time bomb that now is in the face of all attempts at health-care reform.

The Seventies: Growing the Enterprise

Of course, greed was never the stated reason for "usual and customary" pricing under Medicare. Greed is typically sublimated to other forms of self-aggrandizement—serious human failings that don't quite convey the sinfulness of greed. Physicians and surgeons were not leaping to relinquish any control of clinical practice to the government, including its fee-for-service basis. If there was tension within the medical establishment, it related to the existence of group practices like the Health Maintenance Organization (HMO) model Kaiser Health on the West Coast and the private multispecialty clinics in the northern Midwest (Mayo, Gundersen, etc.). Both represented forms of administrative control on private practice. There was even tension with regard to a prepaid health-insurance scheme, the pioneering "HIP" Health Plan founded in New York City in 1947. Ethical concerns were raised by the leadership of the AMA regarding potential abuses, such as "fee splitting," a form of payola for referring patients in network. Advertising was considered unethical. So was interacting with sectarian practitioners, including chiropractors. The medical guild wanted tight control over its purview and its profitability.

"Customary and usual" offered the medical establishment this level of control in the context of Medicare. Medical organizations quickly appreciated the additional sources of income this arrangement provided. Tasks that had been considered part of, even intrinsic to, ordinary practice suddenly became the skillful product of special training and therefore more valuable. Changing dressings, removing sutures, preoperative and postoperative care, and much more became separate tasks, billed separately. Furthermore, a dichotomy took hold. Physicians who attained expertise in procedures or in the application of expensive hardware such as imaging modalities were to be valued over those whose expertise played out solely in the realms of diagnosis and management. The latter are denigrated as members of specialties that are only "cognitive." The dichotomy plagues the structure of the American health-care system to this day.

However, this dichotomy, the AMA leadership, private practitioners, and other advocates of fee-for-service medicine were not the prime movers in the escalation of pricing. Rather, the escalation has resulted more from unintended and unpredicted consequences of Medicare's "usual and customary" compromise. Four stodgy, apolitical, ancillary institutions were the recipients of largesse they never knew to seek in the first place. Each slowly found a way to take advantage so that by the end of the decade, each wielded a great deal of power. This transition required the recruitment of leaders who were comfortable with the language of altruism. Under the guise of altruism, they grew their institutions to become powers unto themselves.

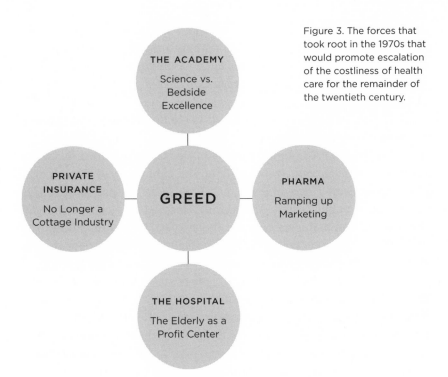

Figure 3. The forces that took root in the 1970s that would promote escalation of the costliness of health care for the remainder of the twentieth century.

The Transition of the Medical School into the Academic Health Center

Prior to World War II, most American medical schools were still home-grown and provincial educational institutions with a sparse full-time faculty staffing the lecture halls and voluntary clinical faculty teaching at the bedside on open wards. The "wards" served the needs of hospitalized charity cases, who in turn served as teaching cases for students and a few "house officers." The latter were postgraduate young physicians who literally lived "in-house," just as many of the nurses lived in the nurses' residence. Most postgraduate training ended with an internship, after which the young physicians marched into general practice and learned to apply unctions and plasters as well as practice obstetrics and perform not-so-minor surgeries. Specialization was exceptional. After all, little in the black bag required detailed knowledge as much as wisdom and experience. Many hospitals had "private" services that catered to the needs of those who could afford more comfort and privacy. They were attended to by their private "attending" doctor and were spared the inconvenience of serving as teaching material.

There were a handful of elite institutions distinctive for faculties of sufficient size that enabled them to commit much of their time to research. These scientists were funded largely from private sources, including their own resources. They were typically men of considerable means. Academic medicine and medical research was a rich man's sport. That changed after the Truman administration created the modern National Institutes of Health.

The history of the National Institutes of Health starts in the nineteenth century with the Laboratory of Hygiene. The Laboratory of Hygiene was part of the Marine Hospital Service and housed a few pioneers of bacteriology and public health. The Marine Hospital Service was charged with serving merchant seamen, particularly with regard to ship-borne epidemics. It was to become the Public Health Hospital system in 1912, which was active into the 1970s. The Laboratory of Hygiene was renamed the National Institute of Health by Congress in the Ransdell Act in 1930. By the end of World War II, the Public Health Service had become a national health agency and the National Institute of Health a research institute that was turning its attention to much more than infectious disease. Harry Truman was president from 1945 to 1953. In 1948 the National Heart Act changed the name of the National Institute of Health to the National Institutes of Health (NIH) and greatly expanded the facilities in Bethesda, Maryland. In 1953 the NIH's research hospital, the Clinical Center, opened on its campus, and the entire Public Health Service, including the NIH, became part of the new Department of Health, Education, and Welfare. That's when the budget took off, exceeding $30 billion by 2012.

The modern NIH is not simply the campus in Bethesda and its intramural research program. Most of its funding, currently well over 80 percent, supports "extramural" programs—that is, the research efforts of scientists at other institutes, most of whom apply for NIH grants for projects they initiate. Some are responding to initiatives developed at the NIH itself. The availability of extramural funding was to change the scope of the research agenda in the country, and not just in terms of topics of interest. It made it possible for medical research to be a viable career option for talented scientists without personal wealth and for medical schools without a research tradition. Today, over 3,000 institutions, mainly schools, institutes, and hospitals affiliated with universities, receive research support by this mechanism.

As important as extramural funding was for the development of medical research nationwide, the modern NIH provided America with an even more valuable gift: scientific talent. A postdoctoral intramural training program was established with funding to support research associates, who would work exclusively in laboratories, and clinical associates, who would staff the Clinical Center and also be assigned to research laboratories. Most on the NIH staff are government employees in the civil service, but some, including the clinical associates, are commissioned officers in the Public Health Service. Some of this change took place in the era of universal military conscription and the Vietnam War "draft." Because of the need for physicians, medical students were exempted from the draft until they completed their first postgraduate (internship) year. The need for specialists, particularly surgeons, was recognized, so the Berry Plan was enacted that exempted some physicians while they were in specialty training programs. There were other needs demanding personnel, including serving the public-health agenda itself by staffing the Public Health Service's Centers for Disease Control (CDC) and the Clinical Center of the NIH. While not considered "military," the Public Health Service is a "uniformed" service whose officers could provide this manpower while satisfying the conscription mandate. Serving two years in this capacity had great appeal to many medical students—so much appeal that an application and rigorous selection process was established. As a result, for many years, clinical associates in the Clinical Center of the NIH were drawn from an applicant pool of the top students from the top medical schools and postgraduate training programs. Many had investigative proclivities and experience; all were exposed to elite science. Some stayed on at the NIH, while most fanned out across the country as faculty members in many medical schools pursuing investigative careers supported by investigator-initiated extramural grants from the NIH.

I was privileged to be part of this ethos. It was a golden age for academic medicine. I was a clinical associate in the Arthritis and Rheumatism Branch of the National Institute of Arthritis and Metabolic Diseases from 1970 to 1972. My clinical duties were the care of patients admitted to the Clinical Center on research protocols designed by investigators in this particular institute. Across the corridor from the patient-care facility were the research laboratories. I was accepted to work in the immunochemistry laboratory directed by Henry Metzger. I had been involved in clinical medicine since early in high school and in scientific research leading to publications starting late in high school. I was no novice. But the experience as a clinical associate took me to another level and did so with an extraordinary peer group. All of us carried the sheen of these golden years with us when we moved on, and many of us understand how commitment, talent, and ethics are necessary to maintain or return such moments to the academy. I look back with great fondness on the decades I enjoyed the pursuit of very basic science in my laboratory surrounded by colleagues and students of like mind and supported by extramural funds from the NIH. My research interests shifted toward clinical epidemiology; if it hadn't, I'd still be poking away at the physical biochemistry of the constituents of bones and joints. Many of my NIH cohort are still so engaged.

Investigator-initiated research grant applications were always competitive. The application is a comprehensive document that is placed before a "Study Section" composed of peers with related research interest. Primary and secondary reviewers present their assessment to other members of the Study Section, who then score the application based on its inherent merit and its merit relative to other applications before the Study Section. Scores that fell below the funding threshold were common, thereby testing the scientific convictions of investigators and their mettle in convincing their institutions to provide "bridge" support for their efforts until they could reapply. Early on, for reasons we will discuss next, such support was often forthcoming. Obtaining funding was never a trivial part of investigative life; today, it is ever more demanding, consuming as much or more creativity and perseverance as the research itself.

That's the investigator's perspective. The perspective of the institutions that house these investigators is not entirely complementary. Research grants from the NIH supported more than the cost of the experiments. It provided the salaries of the personnel, including the principal investigator. And it provided "indirect costs," a payment to the institution housing the research. Indirect costs were a percentage of the direct costs negotiated on an institution-by-institution basis, ranging from around 50 percent to nearly 100 percent of the grant. In other words, if a principal investigator was awarded a grant of $1 million, the institution would get an additional sum to support the work. It became customary for these institutions to generate the funds for research buildings from separate sources (usually private donors and state or federal coffers). The indirect costs paid for the softer infrastructure. It doesn't cost that much to clean and light buildings. The indirect costs fueled the burgeoning of a bureaucracy, often with inflated titles and salaries, designed to manage moneys, process applications, and respond to the proliferation of regulations emanating from a federal research bureaucracy. All sorts of people are involved in monitoring the monitors and regulating the regulators.

This is a vicious cycle. NIH support made it possible for talented scientists to pursue their academic interests. This growing research community created a bureaucracy that depended on "grantsmanship" for its sustenance. The bureaucracy slowly became the tail wagging the dog. "Scholars" were more valued in such a setting for the money they could attract than for the ideas they generated or the students they influenced. The more entrepreneurial the scientist, the more likely he or she was to be rewarded in salary and in influence, including influencing priorities at the NIH, the decisions of Study Sections, and the intellectual climate of their home institutions.

The Creation of the Modern Hospital

While the academic side of the modern predatory academic health center was taking shape as an unintended consequence of post–World War II enlightenment, the clinical side was not ignored. In *The Care of Strangers: The Rise of America's Hospital System* (1987), Charles Rosenberg brilliantly details the history of the growth of the American hospital system up to the mid-twentieth century and its relationship to medical education. In the 1950s, America was dotted with proprietary hospitals, which were usually modest in size and run as private businesses with little oversight at any level. There were also larger and more prominent voluntary hospitals that were supported by private donations and community coffers. Many had private pavilions where the needs of advantaged patients were attended to. Most had "wards" for those who could not afford to pay. Municipal hospitals were often nothing more than sprawling wards—Boston City Hospital, Bellevue in New York, Charity in New Orleans, Grady in Atlanta, Cook County, Hennepin County, and others.

In the late 1960s, I was a student and then a house officer at Massachusetts General Hospital. The institution had three levels of care. Phillips House was so exclusive that only the doctor's name was on the front of the chart to assure patient anonymity. Rooms were private and well-appointed. House officers and students were not assigned to these patients and were not to venture into this sanctum unless requested because of an emergency or other special circumstance. Patients with health insurance were admitted to the Baker Pavilion. These were largely semi-private rooms that would seem customary today. All patients had private physicians. However, this was a "teaching service" too. House officers, usually shadowed by medical students, were assigned to help the private physicians care for their patients. A member of the faculty was assigned to supplement the educational climate by making teaching rounds with these house officers. The centerpiece of clinical education was the Ward Service—the Bullfinch Building for medicine and the White Building for surgery. This was the domain of the house officer, with authority stratified by seniority. Patients were admitted to the "service" and cared for by the residents assigned to the service at the time. Faculty supervised by virtue of "teaching rounds" and other interactions with the residents about the care of their patients. This was an obligation of the faculty for which there was no direct remuneration. But then, there was no fee-for-service collected on the wards.

I could surprise you with a discussion of the advantages for patients on the ward services of elite teaching hospitals. But wards are history. Medicare took care of that. The majority of hospitalized patients are elderly, and none need be wards of the state thanks to Medicare. This fact dramatically altered the financing and the organization of the American hospital. Wards disappeared into the semiprivate pavilions. Furthermore, the treating physician was entitled to customary and usual fees for services. There would still be charity care for younger patients who lacked insurance or other means to pay, but the elderly no longer needed to be beneficiaries of charity care. Room, board, use of facilities, overhead, and much more were "usual and customary" hospital charges underwritten by Medicare.

Suddenly, these institutions enjoyed a steady stream of money. The open wards that typified the Ward Service were replaced by semiprivate rooms, and the absence of a physician of record was history. Furthermore, since there was less of a financial barrier to hospitalizing the elderly, not-for-profit hospitals were generating the liquidity to grow in number, size, and attractiveness to patients of all ages. The small proprietary hospitals were overwhelmed, and they disappeared. They are making a comeback in the twenty-first century as specialty hospitals, but I'm getting ahead of the story.

These not-for-profit hospitals grew more than new beds; they grew administrative overhead. The days of the small executive staff and a purchasing officer or two were gone. Furthermore, the management of the care of the patient was no longer solely the purview of those at the bedside delivering the care. Supervisors and supervisors of supervisors proliferated. Some of this seems the predictable fate of service professions once there is money to grow with. Some of this comes with federal mandates. The federal government has a fiduciary responsibility to assure that its moneys are spent efficiently and effectively. Regulations beget regulations, and regulators require administrators to interact with. Even Medicare billing, the single-payer model of a fee-for-service insurance scheme, rapidly grew in complexity.

Reimbursement is item by item—from dressings to dressing changes, from pill to pill—and that's only for materials. How much should room and board cost? Where do you build in the cost of nursing personnel, pharmaceutical services, and the like? How do you assure that the bills are not spuriously inflated? The answers are in layers of regulations, forms, designations, oversight, and burgeoning bureaucracies in every hospital and in every other practice setting. All this added to the Medicare fee structure, so that you can buy an aspirin in a supermarket for a few pennies but the charge on an in-patient bill is many dollars. A complete blood count is now done by machine for a cost of less than fifty cents, but Medicare is billed for each element that is reported at a cumulative cost of fifty dollars or more.

The pressure to inflate the cost of services spills over to the inflated sense of worth of the administrators of these not-for-profit institutions. They become the superstructure rather than the infrastructure. The running of an organization rendered ever more complex requires more people who consider their skills more valuable than the skill sets required for delivering care itself. By the 1980s, "hospital administration" had evolved from a management track that was neither glamorous nor particularly well paid to a large, visible, lucrative, and sought-after career path. Eyebrows were not raised when someone with an M.D. decided that an MBA would be useful. Eyebrows are not raised when an administrator of a state-supported hospital is paid much more than the governor (though not as much as the football coach).

By the way, does anyone question the source of the moneys that build these shining, marble citadels? The "through put" (flow of profitable "units of care") pays for the feeding and watering of the administration, for those who run the infrastructure, even for some caregivers. But assembling the bricks and mortar is serviced differently. Some institutions still have access to philanthropists who pay for naming rights. Some still have access to the pocketbooks of taxpayers. But many have floated bonds, often tax-exempt "municipal" bonds that appeal to the wealthy as a safe, even insured, income-generating haven for their wealth. However, this means that the hospitals have debt to service. The arrangement is peculiarly American, though other countries are starting down this path. The expense of servicing debt is incorporated into your hospital bill. Isn't this taxation without representation? Would you forego the expansive marble lobby for lesser charges?

What happened to the teaching service in this dialectic? It was agreed that Medicare would pay a higher bed charge in teaching hospitals to cover the salaries of house officers. Prior to this, house officer salaries were meager, barely subsistence. In fact, they were called house officers because traditionally they lived in the hospital, in-house, and generally put off marriage (that was a requirement in many institutions). Thanks to Medicare, salaries increased well beyond subsistence. But it seemed reasonable not to consider the house officer as the doctor of record; that designation fell to the teaching faculty member whenever the patient lacked a private physician. This represented a new income source for faculty, one that could supplant other sources of income relied upon in the past. For teaching faculty on salary, this stream flowed into the coffers of their academic department, and some was, and still is, passed on to the administration of the affiliated medical school as a tithe.

Early on, it was customary for faculty to request no salary for themselves in their NIH grant applications; it was a statement of pride that they were able to volunteer their time for this greater good because their income was secure from clinical sources. That moment of magnanimity was fleeting. Academic physicians and their institutional administrators would craft some sort of partitioning of effort so that one grant might budget 22 percent and another grant 28 percent (or some such) of their time as being committed to the research, and they then prorated the salary request accordingly. This interpretation of faculty fees-for-service hit a Department of Justice wall in 1996. Several august institutions were heavily fined for double-dipping; the federal government cited the practice of piggybacking faculty salaries on top of the moneys for house officer salaries that were incorporated into bed charges. There was brouhaha and then a compromise: if faculty were to be reimbursed as the treating physicians, they must serve each patient independent of the house officers. Clinical education at the bedside in the United States has suffered mightily to preserve this institutional income stream.

Bureaucrats don't understand that. Thanks to Medicare, the numbers on the faculty had escalated, and all were expected to repay their home institution with the moneys they could generate from various sources that would support their salary and then some. The overage nurtured the avarice of the administration. Hence, the clinical side merged with the academic side to form the modern academic health center. All of these unintended consequences of post–World War II enlightenment were costly and resulted in a burgeoning, self-serving infrastructure. But they were not sullying the ethics that fostered Medicare and the modern NIH. The seeds of ethical bankruptcy had been planted, but they didn't really take root in the 1970s. Two other forces had to come into being first.

The Health-Insurance Industry Is Born

As mentioned, very few Americans had health insurance prior to 1960. The insurance industry had expanded greatly in the first half of the twentieth century thanks to the profitability of indemnity plans insuring life, casualty, property, and liability. Health insurance existed but was a minor player with generally local impact. For example, in 1929 Baylor University offered the employees of its health-care facilities in Dallas the option of purchasing a policy that would insure for a limited hospital stay. Several other institutions started offering similar plans, causing the American Hospital Association to set standards in 1939 and adopt the Blue Cross rubric for this agenda. As more plans developed, the Blue Cross Association broke away from the American Hospital Association and became the licensing organization for a growing number of small, independent companies. The first of the Blue Shield plans insuring care by doctors emerged in California in 1939. In 1982 these two industry conglomerations merged to form the Blue Cross Blue Shield Association (BCBS), which has a membership today of some forty independent companies insuring 100 million or so Americans. But in the 1960s, the member companies were just getting off the ground. Some of the older insurance companies were also developing health-insurance lines—companies like Aetna, Connecticut General Life Insurance Company, and the Insurance Company of North America (the last two would merge as Cigna in 1982).

The regulatory precedent for health insurance was the workers' compensation system. Workers' compensation insures employees for medical care and lost wages consequent to a personal injury that occurred while working. When workers' compensation was first proposed in the United States in 1910, the U.S. Supreme Court decided that a federal mandate for such coverage was unconstitutional: it would be a form of taxation without representation, even though the costs were to be borne by employers. (This precedent did not sway the deliberations as to the constitutionality of the 2010 Affordable Care Act.) As a result, the workers' compensation indemnity scheme reverted to the states. It was adopted state by state, with a few federal jurisdictions thrown in. All of these schemes started with a similar template, but each state crafted different regulatory nuances. Since the early health-insurance plans were local, not federal, and since each state already had agencies regulating workers' compensation, state regulation of health insurance followed naturally and continues to do so. Hence, we have a large number of state-based BCBS affiliates, and even the monolithic companies such as Aetna and Cigna have to modify policies on a state-by-state basis.

This is not the only influence of the workers' compensation precedent. It seemed natural for health insurance to follow workers' compensation as a benefit underwritten by employers. This is not to say that employers leaped to assume the cost of the workers' compensation benefit. That cost was passed on to the consumer in the price of goods and services and represented a degree of uncertainty for employers' profit margins. The compromise that enticed American employers was "tort immunity." In exchange for their employer indemnifying wages and health care, the injured worker could not sue the employer for damages unless there was abject malfeasance. There is a parallel aspect to employer-provided private health insurance under the Employee Retirement Income Security Act of 1974 (ERISA). If an employee feels that particular health services were denied inappropriately, ERISA stipulates tortuous steps for appeal and for mounting a civil lawsuit.

The sociopolitical and clinical ramifications of workers' compensation are dissected in one of my previous books, *Stabbed in the Back.* Here, we're examining workers' compensation insurance as the precedent for employer-based health insurance. Workers' compensation policies are expensive. The premiums are adjusted by "experience rating," which means that industries with a history of frequent claims spend as much as 8 percent of wages on these premiums. At the other end of the spectrum, the cost is closer to 2 percent, which is not trivial for industries with small profit margins. In some states, such as Texas, it is lawful to "opt out" and pay injured workers on a case-by-case basis, risking lawsuits if a worker feels cheated. But most states require that all but the smallest of employers cover their workforce under its workers' compensation scheme.

These policies are a profit center for some of the largest private-sector insurance companies, including Liberty Mutual, which was founded to serve this business early in the twentieth century. Several state governments, such as those of Ohio and Washington, require small employers to purchase their policy from a state agency; larger employers can self-insure. For all schemes, whether state based or private, this industry has an "actuarially based" premium schedule, which means the insurance company or state agency prorates its charges to take into account the worst contingency, thereby accumulating sufficient moneys in their coffers to cover any long-term disability expense. The coffers can grow quite impressive unless management invests them poorly (as has happened more than once).

Between experience rating and this actuarial business model, the cost of purchasing workers' compensation policies from these companies and agencies is so substantial that most large private employers have long chosen to "self-insure." But that doesn't mean they avoid dealing with the insurance companies and state agencies. Rather, they turn to them to administer their "self-insurance" plan on a cost-plus basis. This is the same principle that operates in many government agencies, such as the Pentagon. Cost-plus means the employer pays whatever medical and indemnity bills are generated by injured workers to the insurance company, who then disburses the moneys. But the insurance company charges a fixed percentage of the moneys flowing through its coffers as a processing fee. Tucked into this processing fee is profit—often substantial profit that inflates executive salaries and stock value. The self-insured employer, not the coffers of the insurer, is the deep pocket to cover all these expenses. The arrangement is particularly appealing since the employer can defray some of the cost as a tax exemption.

This all makes good business sense for employers, who need not stoke insurance company coffers quite as much as if they simply purchased a policy, and for insurance companies, who have assumed no risk. But there is one glaring caveat. There is no incentive on the part of the insurance companies to limit claims. The more claims and the more complex the claims, the greater the profitability. Since the majority of the expense of workers' compensation policies relate to regional back and arm pain in the workplace rather than to violent injuries, there is no reason for insurance companies to question the basis for considering a backache an injury in the first place. However, there is every financial reason to create an expensive and expansive claims-processing mechanism. As mentioned, *Stabbed in the Back* offers a detailed look at this iatrogenic social contract, emphasizing the notions of causation, disability, and disability determination.

The downsides of the American workers' compensation system are not generally appreciated even today. They were not even discussed in the 1960s and 1970s when employer-sponsored, tax-deductible, fee-for-service private health insurance was sweeping the country. Nearly all large private-sector and governmental employers chose to self-insure. Medicare is an extreme example of self-insurance. The federal government, through its agency the Centers for Medicare and Medicaid Services (CMS), turns to the private sector to administer the Medicare indemnity scheme it has crafted. Smaller employers can turn to brokers or trade agencies to gain a pricing advantage when purchasing policies for themselves and their workers. Aside from the HMOs and similar prepaid schemes, very few policies avoid the private-sector cost-plus providers for processing claims.

There is very little transparency in private-sector health insurance. Usually, there is no valid statement of the "plus" in the cost-plus arrangement since one company's "cost" might be considered another company's "profit." In other words, lots of personal aggrandizement can hide in the "cost" categories of marketing, performance bonuses, patient education, and the like. It's even difficult to comparison shop between providers of health care since few are willing to explain their billing. We know from data such as that presented in Table 4 that far more wealth is at play today in the United States than in any peer country.

What is less appreciated is the time course of this disparity (Figure 4). The escalation and the rising disparity were only simmering in the 1970s; the eruption commenced in the 1980s. The synergy between "usual and customary" fee setting and a "cost-plus" provision of employer-sponsored health insurance found relatively little fodder in the clinical scenario of the 1960s or even the 1970s. The fodder was in every new "advance" to come down the pike afterward. The 1970s were to witness the beginning of the technological miracles of modern medicine. Surgeons, radiologists, and medical interventionalists ventured into body cavities where none had ventured before, from hearts to heads to knees and much in between. Biomedical engineers designed tools for imaging, irradiating, repairing, and replacing that had been the stuff of science fiction for generations. Pharmaceutical chemists designed all sorts of agents to enhance, block, or alter every new biological insight that was forthcoming from the basic science establishment. There was no usual and customary precedent for these innovations. There also was no adequate monitor to validate or deny the claims of efficacy and value that accompanied every putative advance. Many of them, particularly many among the most familiar and most expensive, have proved valueless (see chapters 3 through 5). But the country was and remains blindsided; the fox is in the henhouse. The stakeholders declared their own value and set their own pricing—and we paid.

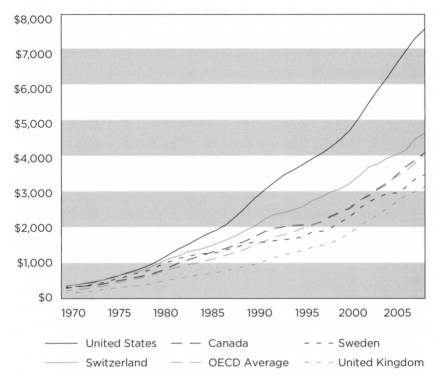

Figure 4. Growth in total health expenditure per capita, United States and selected countries, 1970–2008 (adjusted for purchasing power parity). (Source: Organization for Economic Co-operation and Development [2010], "OECD Health Data," *OECD Health Statistics* [database]; doi: 10.1787/data-00350-en; accessed February 14, 2011)

The Pharmaceutical Industry Casts off
Its Provincial and Primitive Shackles

The pharmaceutical industry before World War II was more colorful than important. No one could have imagined it would become the behemoth that it is today. Most of the companies were pedaling "patent medicines" and pandering to a gullible market that was inclined to ingest potions and concoctions for whatever ailed them, a gullible market that continues to grow by the day. The largest player was an offshoot of the dye industry, which made a fortune pedaling one of the very few effective medicines: aspirin. Aspirin had been synthesized by Karl Löwig by modifying salicin, the poorly tolerated, active principle of willow bark that had been used to treat fever for centuries. Aspirin was one of many synthetic compounds that was gathering dust on the shelves of IG Farbenfabriken in Bayer-

Elberfeld until another chemist, Felix Hofmann, had the temerity to talk his father into trying it for his rheumatism.

This event was not lost on Friedrich Carl Duisberg Jr., who envisioned an entire new market for the chemical industry. Duisberg was another chemist working at the small dye chemical company Friedrich Bayer & Co. When Duisberg got done, he had transformed it into the giant IG Farben, and he had moved Bayer aspirin into the fabric of daily living around the world. The Bayer factory in Rensselaer, New York, opened in 1903 and, along with the Bayer brand and the "Bayer Cross," became a spoil of World War I, coming under the ownership of an American patent-medicine firm that evolved into Sterling Products. The brand returned to Germany in a financial transaction at the turn of the current century. But Duisberg's model of a chemical enterprise creating pharmaceuticals caught on long before there were other effective chemicals to purvey. Bristol-Myers, American Home, and Miles Laboratories (Alka-Seltzer) joined Sterling in evolving from patent-medicine firms into lucrative industrial powerhouses that, early on, were competing among themselves and with IG Farben for the sale of aspirin and aspirin-containing preparations. Aside from aspirin, there were very few triumphs of the pharmaceutical industry before World War II.

Then came antibiotics. The first, Prontisil, was a triumph of IG Farben chemists. Sulfonamidochrysoidine was synthesized by Bayer chemists Josef Klarer and Fritz Mietzsch as part of a research program designed to find dyes that might act as antibacterial drugs in the body. The molecule was patented in Germany; it was then tested and found effective in 1932 against some important bacterial infections in mice by Gerhard Domagk, who subsequently received the 1939 Nobel Prize in Medicine. Prontosil was the result of five years of testing involving thousands of compounds related to azo dyes. Shortly after Prontosil became available in Germany, sulphapyridine was synthesized by the British firm May & Baker, Ltd. It is the miracle drug that was said to have saved Winston Churchill's life in Tunisia in 1943.

The pharmaceutical industry was not the setting for the other great discoveries of antibiotics in this era. Alexander Fleming was a pharmacologist on the staff of St. Mary's Hospital and Medical School in London when he discovered penicillin in 1929. The discovery lay relatively fallow until 1940, when Howard Florey and Ernst Chain at the Radcliffe Infirmary in Oxford purified it sufficiently for clinical trials. All three men shared the Nobel Prize for Medicine in 1945. Selman Waksman was a research microbiologist at Rutgers University interested in fungi in the soil when he discovered streptomycin. He received the Nobel Prize in 1952 for discovering the first antibiotic effective against tuberculosis.

For the following decade, maybe two, the world was advantaged by the symbiosis between scientists working independently in industry and those working in the academy. In fact, the research campuses of the major pharmaceutical firms were often as academic as those in the academy. In both, scientists felt a degree of freedom to pursue their ideas relatively unfettered by financial constraints arising from the need to generate profitable compounds or gain research funding. Gertrude Elion and George Hitchings shared the Nobel Prize in 1988 for ushering novel compounds from the bench to the bedside while working at the Burroughs-Wellcome laboratories in the United States, and John Vane was awarded his Nobel Prize in 1982 for basic scientific discoveries while at the Wellcome Research Laboratories in the United Kingdom.

However, independent scientific thought brings with it many a false start. That means for every success story, there are a legion of hard-working, dedicated scientists who do not enjoy succulent fruits of their labor. That is tolerated in the academy, and valued as long as the work is funded, because these scientists are role models who embody professional dedication and teach others in the methods of pursuing new knowledge. The more the bottom line comes to dominate the enterprise, however, the less the pursuit of knowledge for knowledge's sake is valued. The legendary Wellcome Research Laboratories succumbed to this dialectic. It was no match for the new age pharmaceutical firm. It's a story worth telling.

James Black was a Scottish physician and pharmacologist who discovered propanolol (the prototype beta-blocker, like atenolol) while working in the research laboratories of ICI, a British pharmaceutical firm, between 1958 and 1964. His method was to understand the chemistry of adrenaline and design a compound to specifically block the activity. This was a groundbreaking methodology that he also applied to histamine, a body chemical that causes acid to be secreted in the stomach by attaching to specific receptors. Black designed a molecule to block this reaction too. He pursued this line of research at the British research laboratories of Smith Kline and French (SKF), a Philadelphia-based pharmaceutical firm. The result was cimetidine, the ulcer drug that was released as Tagamet in 1975 and quickly supplanted propanolol as the most prescribed pharmaceutical. James Black received his Nobel Prize in 1988.

Glaxo was a venerable British drug house, meaning it was an imperious establishment enterprise that was nurtured by imperial profitability.

In other words, it had the Raj as its captive market long after dissolution of the empire. But the handwriting was on the wall, and new markets and products had to be developed to survive. In the 1970s, Glaxo established a beachhead in Shreveport, Louisiana, and began purveying Zorprin, a "long acting" aspirin compound that had no rationale to support the aggressive American-style marketing. Then along came ranitidine. John Bradshaw synthesized ranitidine in the summer of 1976 using James Black's methodology. It is chemically and biologically similar to cimetidine but requires less-frequent dosing and may have a slight edge in tolerability. Glaxo quickly found an edge in marketing it as Zantac in 1981; physicians in large numbers found a reason to purchase Glaxo stock, and Glaxo left its stodgy past in the dust. Zantac rapidly climbed to number one in pharmaceutical sales. It was the "blockbuster" drug that changed the corporate philosophy and trajectory. Merger after merger followed, so that Glaxo swallowed Burroughs-Wellcome and SKF to morph into the Anglo-American behemoth GlaxoSmithKline.

This "success" story has been the gold standard for performance in the pharmaceutical industry ever since. The name of the game is the "blockbuster." It is pursued at all cost. Science for the sake of science has no place in this pursuit. The generation of novel ideas can be delegated to the academy and the small start-up firms; once there is promise of a blockbuster, the idea can be co-opted or purchased. The notion of a "blockbuster" goes well beyond the pharmacology of any agent. It is rooted primarily in sales and nurtured by marketing. If the drug really works only in some patients, the goal is to convince doctors and patients that it might work in other patients. If the drug barely works, the goal is to convince doctors and patients that it's worth the try because they might get lucky. To be a blockbuster demands both medicalization and overtreatment in some combination. To be a blockbuster demands convincing a large population that adverse events are a price worth paying. To be a blockbuster demands a license from the FDA that does not squelch the exercise. That requires Phase III randomized controlled trials designed for this purpose (chapter 3).

Just as the pharmaceutical behemoths have outsourced the generating of new ideas, so too were they inclined to outsource these requisite licensing trials. Dennis Gillings will not receive a Nobel Prize, unless there's a new category for entrepreneurship. Dennis and I joined the faculty of the University of North Carolina at the same time in the early 1970s; he entered the Department of Biostatistics in the School of Public Health and I the Department of Medicine in the School of Medicine. We became collaborators, coauthors, and friends. Dennis is a brilliant applied mathematician who was soon sought out by pharmaceutical firms as a consultant on the design of drug trials. These were the early days of the quest for the blockbuster, and Dennis understood the statistical prerequisites instinctively. By 1982 his consulting efforts had become Quintiles Transnational, the first Contract Research Organization (CRO). As documented in chapter 1, Quintiles Transnational has grown to employ over 20,000 people and to generate over $3 billion in annual revenues. It now sits atop a large new industry to which the pharmaceutical firms of all sizes turn for the design and execution of drug trials and the negotiation of the maze to licensure by the FDA. The quest for a blockbuster demands designing trials that permit one to extrapolate to a large population of potential consumers. This opens the door to all the abuses we discuss in other chapters—abuses in patient recruitment, in data analysis, in extrapolation, and in the use of surrogate outcomes. It opens the door to the creation of "trialists" and "thought leaders" and other physicians who have to contend with conflictual relationships with the CRO and the contracting pharmaceutical firm. In fact, the notion of a CRO is inherently conflictual. It is contracted to test for efficacy rather than to try to disprove efficacy. The latter is sound science. The former is profitable.

Speaking of profitable, the free market is no match for pharmaceutical pricing. First, newly licensed drugs are patented. That grants exclusive rights to the manufacture and sales of the pharmaceutical for twenty years from the filing date. This elimination of free-market competitiveness is one of the arguments for "me too" pharmaceuticals. These are drugs that are dissimilar enough to justify a separate patent but similar in terms of efficacy. The argument hardly holds water since "me too" pharmaceuticals tend to be marketed aggressively for their marginal differences rather than for any cost savings. All drugs on patent in the United States are priced on average 50 percent higher than they are in the European Union and higher yet than in Japan (which leads the world in per capita consumption of prescription pharmaceuticals). The industry defends its pricing structure as necessary to cover the expenses of drug development. The argument is hardly convincing—and not just in light of executive compensation packages, bottom-line profitability, and stock prices. Much that is called "drug development" is marketing dressed up for public-relations purposes. That includes the "seed trials" discussed in chapter 1, which are CRO exercises in pseudoscience designed to enhance familiarity with drugs rather than to test important hypotheses.

Reining in the Beast Is Creating the Monster

Mark Hall and Carl Schneider have written an elegant essay on the history of billing for medical fees in Western society ("Learning from the Legal History of Billing for Medical Fees," *Journal of General Internal Medicine* 23, no. 8 [2008]: 1257–60). Fee-for-service is a modern innovation. Physicians in antiquity had a "public calling" and relied on the voluntary payment of an "honorarium" as a fee. This is a form of noblesse oblige that set professionalism above commercialism. It maintains a foothold in Europe to this day, but it did not cross the Atlantic to the American colonies. The American notion was that a physician's "public calling" did not exclude choosing who and why to serve, nor did it shy away from being paid for that service.

The principles were entrenched in civil law by the twentieth century. The AMA Code of Medical Ethics has stated since 1923 that a "physician is free to choose whom he will serve." The compromise with the principle of a "public calling" was a "sliding scale": the physician determined how much a service was worth and how much a patient was able and willing to pay for any particular service. In 1957 the AMA Code of Medical Ethics required physicians' fees to be "commensurate with the services rendered and the patient's ability to pay." The sliding scale was susceptible to market pressures. Terms such as "charity care," "what the traffic will bear," and "soaking the rich" found their way into parlance and into lawsuits over the reasonableness of fees. Many a general practitioner lived by the sliding scale in the 1960s. But the sliding scale did not survive much longer. The responsibility for "charity care" reverted to public institutions, including the "ward" services of municipal hospitals and the like. Medicare and Medicaid superseded the sliding scale for those who qualified, and the range of private-indemnity schemes substituted for the sliding scale for all others. There was no allusion to a sliding scale in the 1980 revision of the AMA Code of Medical Ethics.

By 1970 all the pieces and players were assembled for the American health-care system to become more a cash cow (Figure 3) than a service profession. It has today become a herd of cash cows, particularly in the United States (Figure 4). The seeds of the trend were in the "reasonable cost" clause of the Medicare legislation. No longer was a sliding scale of fees-for-services supporting a cottage industry. The government and large employers were the de facto consumers of services. The compromise with the AMA to permit "usual and customary" fee-for-service charges is embodied today in yet another new age industry dedicated to defining "service" and setting "fee." In 1966 the AMA first published Current Procedural Terminology (CPT), a set of codes designed to standardize billing for "Evaluation/Management Services" (E/M). The CPT Editorial Panel currently meets three times a year and releases new editions each October to reflect changes in practice. The current version lists numerical codes for more than 10,000 procedures and services.

CPT is the most widely utilized medical nomenclature in reports to public and private health-insurance programs in the United States. In 1983 it was mandated for all billing under Medicare and Medicaid. CPT is also a profitable proprietary undertaking for the AMA, which sells all sorts of educational and other aids to assist in the coding exercise. After all, hospitals and physicians need to be able to accurately code for E/M services or they risk loss of income or fraudulent billing accusations. "Coding" is a burgeoning job category that appeals to many, even to many in the nursing profession. There are courses offered in coding in all sorts of venues, including many junior colleges. Coders are checking on coders, and physicians are admonished if they do not "document" in their records for the sake of coding; they are less likely to be admonished if the content of the record communicates poorly about actual patient care. In fact, coding and billing are driving the design of the Electronic Health Record (EHR) in America. There is no reproducible evidence that the EHR decreases medical errors or increases compliance with "standards" for quality of care. Rather, the purveyance and servicing of EHR has joined coding as yet another profitable industry.

Although the costliness of health care had yet to take off (Figure 4), the inefficiency of paying usual-and-customary fees for each and every coded item was obvious early on, particularly for Medicare and Medicaid patients treated in hospital. It made more sense to pay a lump sum for a particular package of care, a "product" such as a total hysterectomy or an appendectomy. In the 1970s, the Health Care Finance Administration (HCFA), the predecessor agency to the CMS, contracted Robert Fetter, Ph.D., and John Thompson, Ph.D., of Yale's School of Management and School of Public Health, respectively, to create a classification of such "products." The result was 467 Disease-Related Groups (DRGs), the last of which was the "ungroupable" category. The intent was to replace cost-based hospital reimbursement with a prospective payment system based on a presumably homogeneous unit of care.

The system was tested in New Jersey between 1980 and 1983, after which it was adopted by the CMS. Many states have since passed legislation requiring the application of DRG-based billing to privately indemnified hospital care. As a prospective payment system, it was designed to provide incentives for efficient and standardized care. If the patient can be treated in hospital for a particular DRG at a cost less than the prospective payment, the hospital can keep the excess. But if the cost exceeds the allotment, the hospital eats it. Given the proliferation of procedures and the complexity of illnesses, the number of DRGs had escalated to 999 by 2007. Much of this relates to provisos for particularly complex or complicated "products." By hook or by crook, coding was to make sure that the hospital continued to eat well enough to thrive. In 2008 the CMS declared that it would not cover all hospital-acquired conditions, particularly those deemed avoidable. This is a significant stride forward for competent care, since any degree of incompetence leads to codes that change the DRG in a direction that compromises the profitability of the not-for-profit hospital.

The DRG classification takes advantage of an internationally accepted system of disease classification that has its roots in the nineteenth century. The modern version is called the International Statistical Classification of Diseases and Related Health Problems (ICD), which is published by the World Health Organization (WHO) and widely used in the collection of mortality statistics and the like. The ninth edition, the ICD-9, allows for some 17,000 diagnostic categories and is used by the U.S. National Center for Health Statistics, which was instrumental in its development. The ICD-10 has been used since the mid-1990s—but not by the CMS, which adopted it only in the spring of 2013. ICD-10 is a classification system that allows for 155,000 different codes. One can well imagine how the proliferation of ICD codes will beget a proliferation of DRGs. The proliferation of codes is not simply a reflection of the proliferation of disease categories; some of the codes speak to the degree of severity and of complications. ICD-10 coding makes CPT coding look like child's play. Hence, billing according to DRGs is a monumental task for all involved. Hospitals employ minions to find any nuance that might increase the complexity of the basic DRG in order to increase payment. The CMS outsources this billing to employ minions in the exercise of validating the charge package.

How much should any particular DRG cost? That brings us back to the "usual and customary" and "reasonable cost" roots. The hospital and hospital-supply industries are powerful and spared from most of the pressures of a true free market; they operate with a conspiratorial form of the "free market." The same consumable or piece of equipment purchased from a laboratory supply house by an NIH-supported research laboratory can cost multiples more when purchased from a hospital supply house. The competition is set at a different level. The same is true for hospitals. Most hospitals will not publish their fee scale for room maintenance, nursing, and hospital services (such as X-rays or the running of operating rooms). Individual hospitals negotiate this fee schedule with individual private insurance companies. The hospital industry negotiates with the CMS, with provisions for the differences in cost in different geographic regions and with the help of lots of solicited and unsolicited "advice." By law, hospitals must "accept" what the CMS pays even if it is less than their menu of prices for private insurers. Private insurance contracts have no such stipulation. Private insurers pass any bill in excess of the amount charged on to the patient. It's a cozy arrangement that goes to great lengths to avoid transparency. There are even companies that help patients sort through their bills with the intent of finding overcharges that inflate co-pays. There is absolutely no doubt that this cozy arrangement is part of the explanation for the discrepant curves in Figure 4; the other part is overtreatment in the first place.

The best window into this cozy arrangement is the establishment of physician fees by the CMS. In the early 1990s, the CMS turned to the AMA for assistance with fine-tuning physician fees. This seems a logical extension of the role of the AMA in formulating CPTs. The AMA was to set aside "usual and customary" in favor of a new approach to a fair and accurate valuation of procedures and treatments by physicians. This approach was created by William Hsiao, professor of economics at the Harvard School of Public Health, and his multidisciplinary team of colleagues in the mid-1980s. They formulated and tested their Resource-Based Relative Value Scale (RBRVS) and submitted it to HCFA in 1988. In 1989 President George H. W. Bush signed the Omnibus Budget Reconciliation Act stipulating that the CMS base physician payments on the RBRVS. For every code in CPT, a fee was to be determined based nearly equally on physician experience and practice expense (recently, a dollop more was prorated for malpractice insurance). This is where the input of the AMA was sought. In 1991 the AMA established the Specialty Society RBRVS Update Committee (RUC) to advise the CMS as to the value of physician work and practice expense for the physicians providing any particular management/evaluation service coded in CPT.

The RUC has twenty-nine members; twenty-three are appointees of major medical and surgical specialty professional societies and three are AMA appointees. All members sign confidentiality agreements before each meeting, which are closed to the public. The task is to calculate the Relative Value Units (RVU) for each CPT. Since the RUC is specialist dominated and heavily weighted to interventionalists, the RVU calculation is biased to value skills gained by lengthy training and the performance of tasks thought to be "stressful." Cognitive specialties are given short shrift in this calculation. Furthermore, the process values effort over effect, which is contrary to the principles of evidence-based medicine. The incentive is to train to do more, even if the doing is ineffective. There is no incentive to be expert in informing medical decision making, particularly if the informing results in a patient's desire to forego something with a high RVU. There is no incentive for higher quality performance or for caring for the more severely afflicted. RVUS are a perverse measure.

As is true of most areas of administration of the American health-care system, there is little transparency in the machinations that influence the CMS. That means there is little public debate. However, there is debate and controversy among the cognoscenti. The primary-care physicians who are not well represented on the RUC (except for the current AMA-appointed chair) and the cognitive specialists who are in the minority are crying foul. They want to be better valued. I am crying foul because this is an example of a public regulatory agency being controlled by the interests it is meant to regulate. The economists call this regulatory capture. I call it corrupt.

The CMS is a Tower of Babel that is superimposing one flawed remedy upon another in an attempt to rein in the ever-more-unconscionable American benefit/cost ratio. RVUS are a smoke screen. The CMS starts out with charges that are established by specialists and specialty societies as "usual and customary." These charges are two to four times Medicare rates (though private insurers may not balk to this degree). Providers collect 50 to 80 percent of their charges, depending on RVUS and local contractual arrangements. It's smoke and mirrors.

The House of Cards

The Commonwealth Fund is nearly a century old. It was founded by Anna Harkness and charged with the mission of improving health-care practice and policy. Anna Harkness was the widow of Stephen Harkness, a Cleveland entrepreneur who invested with John D. Rockefeller and ended up the second-largest shareholder in Standard Oil. Anna Harkness left enduring marks on the physical plants of Yale, Harvard, and Columbia Universities. But with the Commonwealth Fund, she influenced the development of health policy and its practitioners in the United States and abroad in ways that endure to the present day. One of its influential roles is the issuing of reports that publish health-related data with obvious policy ramifications.

In November 2011, the Commonwealth Fund issued a report detailing the trends in private employer-based health-insurance premiums and deductibles state by state between 2003 and 2010 (http://www .commonwealthfund.org/Publications/Issue-Briefs/2011/Nov/State -Trends-in-Premiums.aspx?omnicid=20). One of the major findings was that the total annual premiums for family coverage increased 50 percent across the country in that period. Employers have been passing more and more of this cost on to their employees, so that the amount the employee contributed directly to premium cost increased over 60 percent. The cost of the policies would be even greater if it were not for deductibles. Deductibles are the annual sum the insured must pay before insurance kicks in. Per-person deductibles doubled over this period. If premiums continue to rise at this rate, the average premium for family coverage will rise to nearly $24,000 by the end of the decade, with deductibles rising apace.

We don't have to wait until 2020 to feel the pain, however. Already over 60 percent of Americans under age sixty-five live where health-insurance premiums are over 20 percent of their income. In 2010 the average private-employer premium for family coverage was nearly $14,000, the average employee contribution for family coverage was nearly $4,000, and deductibles averaged nearly $2,000. In addition, larger employers are required to provide workers' compensation insurance for their workforce at an expense that ranges between 2 percent and 8 percent of salary depending on the industry and the location. Private employers are parsing some $20,000 per employee for "health care." Several years ago, I was invited to convene a seminar for select senior management at Cigna's home office near Hartford, Connecticut. Cigna itself is a private employer and shares the pain of health-care coverage for its sizeable workforce. Of course, I am less concerned about Cigna's pain since it serves its stable of large employers with a form of cost-plus contract; the more money flowing through the system, the larger the sum that the insurance company takes off the top. And these insurance companies are doing well for themselves and in blunting any competitive pressures. In thirty-four states and the District of Columbia, over 70 percent of the health-insurance business has been captured by three or fewer companies. Oregon, Kansas, Wisconsin, and West Virginia are the only states where the majority of the health-insurance market is captured by more than three companies.

Like it or not, depending on whether you are paying or are paid, the current approach to health care merits several descriptions, among which "unsustainable" is the most charitable. Furthermore, the current approach to "reform" incorporates many of the present features that render it unsustainable and perverse. That's because too few Citizen Patients realize that most of the unsustainable features are also the most perverse.

3

Truth and Consequences

MARKETING WITH
TORTURED AND MASSAGED DATA

In chapter 1, "Shills," I used the example of the marketing of Crestor to illustrate several of the ways that science can be corrupted to serve masters with agendas other than truth, let alone improving the care of patients. But there are many ways that scientific methods and scientific results can be bent to such ends. There is nothing new about this potential. Epistemologists of every ilk, not just philosophers of science, have been hard at the task of unraveling scientific missteps, whether intentional or not, for millennia. Nonetheless, egregious practices persist because they are dressed up in the misconceptions and preconceived notions of successive generations. They remain common and are becoming ever more commonplace. Citizen Patients can decry the trend only if they learn to recognize these practices. This chapter is written to cement such an awareness and to teach the skills necessary for identifying health-care deceptions. How do we discern which assertions about our health, or lack thereof, are simply fatuous or just untenable on scientific grounds? How do we discern the degree to which we might benefit from medical assertions that have survived scientific testing? Formulating a theory as to the cause or cure of any of life's many predicaments is not the challenge; knowing which theory is testable requires a degree of genius. Testing the theory requires training, perseverance, and honesty. But understanding the need to separate the wheat from the chaff by demanding clarity cannot be delegated to "authority" alone any longer, if it ever could. A Citizen Patient must be prepared to listen actively and effectively to the explanation.

I have more than a passing interest in epistemology. I am not a professional philosopher, but I am a physician, and every physician should be a philosopher in the classical sense of one who values wisdom. Unfortunately, for much of its history, medicine engaged in the quest for a philosopher's stone, claiming success after success, while great philosophers—epistemologists such as David Hume, John Stuart Mill, and Karl Popper—considered why such a quest and why such claims might be foolhardy. The philosopher's stone was a mythical medieval substance capable of an array of marvels, from turning base metals into gold to curing disease and even prolonging life indefinitely. It was an example of magical thinking that captured the belief systems of many for centuries, including the likes of Sir Isaac Newton. Much that medicine proclaimed to be marvelously curative prior to the middle of the twentieth century was the stuff of the philosopher's stone, marvels that faded away and were superseded by others destined to fade. A few from antiquity, such as colchicine for gout, survive. But few since have proved durable. Drugs that induce anesthesia and techniques for repairing some wounds are exceptions. Most marvels were relegated to archives for subsequent generations to deride.

Durable marvels are a legacy of post–World War II medical science. There are many examples, from penicillin to kidney dialysis. Nonetheless, much that is considered clinically marvelous today is the stuff of the philosopher's stone. These marvels are no longer clothed in the metaphysical idioms of ages past. They hide in the language of contemporary theory, theory that seems to ring true to some or most among us. For medicine, theory has always been couched in scientific terms, so that theory today has a far richer glossary available to it than ever before, a glossary that expands almost daily. The degree to which the theory seems compelling reflects the number of credentialed proponents who declare it sensible. If the proponents are in the mainstream, the theory is deemed peer reviewed and peer accepted and is likely to make its way rapidly into the common sense, taking advantage of all the mechanisms we discussed in the prior chapters. The theory then becomes a socially constructed truth that recruits adherents and promotes acceptable actions. If the proponents of the theory are not in the mainstream, the theory is deemed "alternative," and its proponents are deemed sectarian practitioners who recruit fellow travelers to the self-serving task of defying the sanctioned truth. Until the mid-twentieth century, this was the state of Western medicine. It still is today, but now there are powerful forces of enlightenment working to push medicine off the philosopher's stone. These are the forces that demand we call a theory a theory. If the theory can't be tested, it is nothing but theory. If it can be tested, it should be.

Throughout history, there have been physicians who were uncomfortable with the philosopher's stone and with the empirical medicine by trial and error that it fostered. Even in antiquity, some called for a more scientific approach based on establishing efficacy before unleashing the marvel du jour. There has been no more clarion a call than that articulated about 1,000 years ago by Avicenna, a Persian physician who looms large in the medical pantheon. He authored *The Canon of Medicine*, which served as the authoritative textbook not only in the caliphates but in Europe well into the Middle Ages. One chapter was titled "The recognition of the strengths of the characteristics of medicines through experimentation." There are documented instances of such experimentation in the centuries that followed, but they are few and far between, generally involving the determination that a particular substance was toxic. Most had little influence in their time or since. There are instances to the contrary, some quite dramatic because they influenced world history. For example, until James Lind's eighteenth-century experiment, the British navy was at a great disadvantage in the colonial era. Lind demonstrated that those British sailors ("Limeys") whose diets were supplemented with limes were spared scurvy—the often lethal consequence of vitamin C deficiency—and could survive longer at sea.

The randomized controlled trial (RCT) was conceived in its current form around the time of World War II and employed by the British to assess the efficacy of a drug used to treat rheumatoid arthritis. Such an undertaking required epidemiologists and statisticians to develop the methodological wherewithal to test for efficacy. But this effort was somewhat marginalized until the 1960s, when realpolitik forced it into the mainstream of scientific enquiry. The catalyst came in the form of legislation amending the regulations that defined the agenda of the FDA. No longer was the FDA only to monitor the purity and toxicity of drugs; efficacy was added to the prerequisites for licensure of pharmaceuticals. This legislation was not testimony to prescience; it was in response to the thalidomide tragedy. Society learned the hard way that a new pill for the nausea of pregnancy could damage the unborn child. The RCT and all it represents is a presence that molds clinical judgment and informs patient consent. Without its influence, or by ignoring its influence, medicine reverts to the philosopher's stone. Without an appreciation of this, the Citizen Patient is at risk of being uninformed.

The Crucial Difference between Efficacy and Effectiveness

The science of efficacy tests the hypothesis that a particular intervention works in a particular group of patients. The science of effectiveness tests the hypothesis that a particular intervention works as it is generally used in practice where patients are more heterogeneous than those recruited into a RCT. Comparative effectiveness research (CER) asks whether an intervention works better than other interventions in practice. In the summer of 2009, President Barack Obama signed the American Recovery and Reinvestment Act into law. The legislation charged the Institute of Medicine with defining CER. Its Committee on Comparative Effectiveness Research Prioritization rapidly came up with the following: CER is "the generation and synthesis of evidence that compares the benefits and harms of alternative methods to prevent, diagnose, treat, and monitor a clinical condition, or to improve the delivery of care. The purpose of CER is to assist consumers, clinicians, purchasers, and policy makers to make informed decisions that will improve health care at both the individual and population levels." The legislation specifically disallows the extension of CER to cost-effectiveness. That is unconscionable in the American profit-driven medical marketplace.

The Committee on Comparative Effectiveness Research Prioritization elicited over 2,500 opinions from 1,500 stakeholders and produced a list of the 100 highest-ranked topics for CER (www.iom.edu/cerpriorities). Tucked into the legislation was $1.1 billion to support CER. Proposals to undertake CER are now pouring forth from investigators across the land. There is no doubt that an enormous amount of data will be generated by 2015. But there is every reason to doubt whether many inferences can be teased out of these data that will actually advantage patients, consumers, or the health of the nation. The Citizen Patient needs a prepared mind to find the nuggets in the wash of pronouncements.

The gold standard of efficacy research is the randomized controlled trial. In an RCT, a study population is recruited and randomly assigned to receive the study intervention or a comparator, either an intervention with known efficacy or a placebo. RCTs usually monitor carefully defined populations for a limited time, often a year or less. Many diseases of interest are chronic, so that one cannot expect dramatic changes in the short term. Rather than prolong the trials, two compromises are commonly employed: the study population is increased so that one stands a chance of detecting changes in the short term that occur in only a few; and subtle changes that one believes portend dramatic changes in the future are detected and documented. Fiddling with the size of the study population to this end is termed "power considerations" in epidemiology speak. The subtle changes that portend dramatic changes are termed "surrogate measures."

Modern biostatistics has probed every nuance of the RCT paradigm. The result is a highly sophisticated understanding of its limitations, including the degree to which any result might generalize to other sorts of patients. One of the inviolate tenets is that the hypothesis that is tested in any RCT must be established and stated prior to commencing the trial. These trials can produce a tremendous amount of data. For example, one might have tested a primary hypothesis regarding efficacy of a new drug in a large number and array of patients and be unable to discern a difference in a particular outcome between those on the active drug and those on a placebo. That's disappointing. One might be tempted to dissect the population of subjects and ask if there is efficacy in young or old, black or white, male or female, those with a high blood pressure and those with normal blood pressure, etc. You can reanalyze the data stratified in this way, but any difference you find is not definitive. This is called a secondary or exploratory analysis, and at best it generates new hypotheses. The reason it is not definitive relates to the notion of statistical significance: if you go back to the data 100 times, you expect to find an effect five times by chance alone. The limitations of exploratory analyses are well known, but so is the propensity of investigators to proclaim their secondary findings with a vigor designed to fool the reader and the listener.

The predominate methodology employed for CER is a form of secondary analysis. CER is not constrained by limits on patient variability in the recruitment of subjects, as in RCTs. CER utilizes real-world data sets to deduce benefit/harm in a range of patients—including those who might reasonably be excluded from an RCT. This entails large clinical and administrative networks to provide data. Data sets must be large enough to capture individuals' differences that affect the estimates of benefit/harm across the gamut of insurance, age, comorbidities, and lifestyle. This inclusivity is paramount. For example, when we buy a book at Amazon .com, we are given a list of "other books bought by those who bought your book." There is a data-mining program in the background that links characteristics of the book you bought to characteristics of books bought like yours and to the characteristics of buyers. A different list of book recommendations results based on variations in buyer characteristics, such as age, gender, and purchase history. This is analogous to what CER promises. Of all the different types of patients who in theory might benefit from a particular drug or procedure, which age, gender, degree of illness, etc., marks the appropriate subset?

The principle may be the same, but the analytic demands are like night and day between book buying and health-care provisions. In book buying, there is one objective outcome: the book. Health-care outcomes are neither homogeneous nor always objective. The result can differ if the outcome of interest is longevity, function, employment, or aspects of the quality of life. One of the fundamental problems with attempts to rationalize health care is that we still don't agree on how to measure health or rational care. Mining the data without a definition of the outcome we seek is unlikely to come up with insights that are durable, reproducible, and compelling. For CER to be a valid "Amazon" for health care, it has to define and capture the nuances of health-care outcomes and of health-care provision across all sites of care (including the home).

Clearly, any inference regarding relative benefits and harms from the analysis of large data sets is suspect. Shortcomings relating to benefits, harms, and provision of care are lurking. Any statistical modeling would require assumptions and compromises. Hence, the validity of interpreting observational data will depend on the degree to which diagnosis, clinical course, interventions, coincident diseases, personal characteristics, or outcomes is assumed and not quantified. No matter how compulsively this is done, CER demands judgments about the importance of each of these variables. As an example, total knee replacement (TKR) has at present escaped efficacy testing. How would we learn from observational research if TKR works? Some of the relevant variables to assess efficacy can be parsed from observational data such as patient demographics, type of hardware, comorbidities, and the like. However, some variables are very difficult to parse in the best of circumstances, such as a definition of benefit, surgical experience, or—even more elusive—surgical skillfulness.

Therefore, CER alone cannot be the engine of health-care decision making. There is no way to mine the data from practice settings and assume that anything works. One runs the risk of doing comparative ineffectiveness research. Any attempt to compare outcomes must start with a comparator that is known to work, even if it works only in a particular subset. Hence, CER is the cart and efficacy is the horse. The challenge is to define efficacy trials such that the anchoring comparator is clearly efficacious. There are two ways forward. First, we could design efficacy trials that are efficient in providing gold standards across a wider range of patient characteristics. To accomplish this, we would have to expand trials to larger populations and restrict outcome measures to something statistically significant and clinically interpretable, even if that took a great deal of time to observe. And we'd have to foreswear using the data to test any hypothesis that was not established a priori. As just stated, secondary or exploratory analyses that test multiple hypotheses after the fact are bound to find some association just on the basis of chance.

There is a second approach that is more straightforward. We can design elegant RCTs seeking a statistically significant outcome that is not merely interpretable but large enough to be a clinically meaningful, important outcome for the highly selected patient population that was recruited into the trial. The larger the outcome one seeks, the fewer the subjects and the shorter the trial. If no meaningful outcome is detected, we can either abandon the intervention or choose another highly selected population to study. If a clinically meaningful difference is detected, the result can serve as the anchoring comparator for CER. Then one can look at groups of patients in practice and ask if any group does as well or better than the group that was benefited in an important way in the efficacy trial.

Declaring an outcome to be clinically meaningful is the philosophical challenge in the design of efficacy trials. How much effect need we observe in a given patient to feel that intervening was worthwhile? The effect bar is specific to the particular condition being treated. For metastatic cancer, will we raise our eyebrows if life is prolonged by a month, or six months, or a year, or five years? Once this is established, how often must the intervention prove that effective? Or how much more frequently must we see such a good result in the patients treated with the active intervention compared to those exposed to a placebo? This is the absolute difference in outcome frequency.

How high should we set the bar for this absolute difference to consider the results of the trial compelling for using the intervention in all comers who are similar to the subjects in the trial? One way to think about this is to convert the absolute difference between the active intervention and the referent or control into a more intuitive measure: the number needed to treat (NNT). For example, if the outcome is easily measured, such as death or stroke, we might find an intervention valuable if we had to treat twenty patients for some reasonable interval to spare one. Few students of efficacy would be persuaded if we had to treat more than fifty to spare one. Between twenty and fifty delineates debate; smaller effects are ephemeral and subject to false-positive assertions. For an outcome that is more difficult to measure than death or stroke, such as symptoms or quality of life, we might argue for a more stringent bar. If this stringency was applied in the future to the design of RCTS, trials would be more efficient and reliable. Fewer subjects and shorter trial durations would be necessary to test hypotheses that have large absolute differences that are considered meaningful. We'll return to this consideration repeatedly in the chapters that follow so that it will become second nature by chapter 7, where it is seen to be pivotal in the design of any rational health-insurance scheme.

Secondary analysis is not the only aspect of the interpretation of the results of RCTS that is commonly abused—often intentionally by parties that want us to be more impressed with results than can be justified by the science. Forewarned is not just forearmed; it is reason for the Citizen Patient to rally in outrage at such practices. Let's start with the fore-warning.

Why Not Go for It?

Americans pride themselves on their cussed determination, can-do attitude, and fortitude against odds. A "stiff upper lip" is not an appealing option. Many moments in our history bear witness to our determination, some that we are wont to overlook or forget. We are a people who will seek the grail given an opportunity and a reasonable chance of success. This attitude colors our medical decision making.

Let's take lung cancer as an object lesson. There is no licensed drug and no sanctioned regimen for the treatment of metastatic lung cancer that offers the average person more than a few months of survival advantage. That is the conclusion of the relevant RCTS. It is also the objective rationale for offering intervention and for accepting treatment. As I illustrate in *Rethinking Aging*, the choice to demur on the difficulties and challenges of treatments with such limited yield and opt for support and palliation is certainly reasonable. But rationality is not a constant companion in situations that are perceived as desperate. Although all one can reasonably hope for is months of prolonged life, the caring community and the media are likely to point to the exceptional patient who survived years after such treatment. Furthermore, it is understandable that the exceptional survivor and the survivor's oncologist share a sense of triumph. What patient with metastatic lung cancer won't imagine that such a happy outcome awaits them if they agree to treatment? Wouldn't those who care about that patient surge to the cause of treatment and revere those who care for the patient as saviors? Likewise, what pall would surround the decision to respond, "Thanks, but no thanks"? This is not informed decision making. This is an example of a misunderstanding fueling social pressure—of the lottery mentality gone awry.

I don't buy lottery tickets. True, someone will win, and likely win a mind-boggling windfall. That someone may be one in a million, but someone will win. It is so unlikely to be that someone that maybe there's a magical force at play, maybe a gambler's gryphon or a good fairy. Many reasonable Americans must believe in the gambler's gryphon. Some have premonitions, a sense that the gryphon will fend for them in the deepest reaches of improbability where the power ball hides. None of this is irrational behavior. All lottery participants understand the probabilities, and many get a kick out of the possibilities. However, the psychology of the lottery has been so well inculcated that it commonly makes sense to apply it to another challenging win-lose exercise: betting on our health. It drives the "I know the chance is slim, Doc, but let's go for it" response when we or our loved ones are sick. It also drives our choice of a health-insurance plan, as we'll discuss in following chapters. In the case of the lottery, we know what we're doing. In the case of winning good health, we are all too often bamboozled.

The lottery and medical decision making that's informed by an RCT have nothing in common. In the case of the lottery, the chances of winning may be slim, but they are zero if you don't buy a ticket. The RCT answers the question, how much more likely am I to "win" if I take the intervention than I am to "win" if I don't take the intervention? The informative answer is usually expressed in terms of the absolute difference in average improvement from which an NNT can be derived. However, average is one mathematical description of the distribution of responses of the population of subjects in the study. Some do very poorly, and some do exceptionally well in both the treated and the control populations. When you hear that there is the occasional patient who did exceptionally well on the drug for lung cancer in the RCT, suppress your lottery mentality. Ask how likely you are to do exceptionally well if you don't undergo the treatment. When the absolute difference in the average response is not impressive, the answer is that you're almost as likely to do exceptionally well if you don't undergo treatment as if you do. It's like winning the lottery without buying a ticket. And before you say, "OK, I understand, but I can't stand not actively going for this tiny theoretical advantage," ask what the experience of the treatment is like and decide whether any downside of the treatment is worth a run at a remote advantage.

I used lung cancer for our object lesson because it is a desperate circumstance that captures our attention. But marketing can and does play havoc with our rationality by taking advantage of our lottery mentality in far-less-desperate circumstance. The marketing for disease prevention is ripe with such mind games. I'll mention two examples from the several we will discuss in detail in chapter 5.

TREATING HIGH CHOLESTEROL

Let's assume you are a perfectly well middle-aged man who learns that his cholesterol is above the level some committee defined as normal. Now you're worried. You have a "risk factor" for heart disease, stroke, and death before your time. Naturally, you feel relieved that your doctor can pummel your cholesterol below the upper limits of normal if you take her favorite statin drug. Few can refuse. Even fewer pause to wonder whether the result of doing so is meaningful to them. It turns out that if I treat 100 men with a statin and 100 with a placebo, after five years, ninety-six would be alive in both groups. Of the four who died in each group, two died of a heart attack. I wonder if these men would be as worried about their "high cholesterol" if they knew that their risk of death was 2 percent in five years with or without treatment. Of the ninety-six still alive and taking a statin, four had survived a heart attack. Of the ninety-six still alive on placebo, six had survived a heart attack. So if 100 men swallow a statin every day for five years, two might be spared the experience of a nonfatal heart attack. That is a surprisingly meager "win" for swallowing 1,800 pills.*

Here's where the lottery mentality leads us astray. The odds of winning a lottery are orders of magnitude less than 2 percent, yet many go for the win, and someone will win. But the 2 percent reduction in risk of a nonfatal heart attack on a statin does not guarantee anyone will win. In a randomized controlled trial, 2 percent is right on the cusp of irreproducibly

---

* This example is borrowed from the classic "West of Scotland" Trial (*New England Journal of Medicine* 333 [1995]: 1301–7), which is held up to this day as the support for treating well people with statins to prevent heart disease, i.e., primary prevention of heart disease. Even this meager effect did not reproduce in a larger American trial, the ALLHAT-LHT (*Journal of the American Medical Association* 288 [2002]: 296–307).

and therefore unbelievably small. Such small differences often do not re-produce when the trial is repeated. That means you do almost as well on the placebo, and maybe just as well. That's how you can win the lottery without buying a ticket. When the effect size is very small on a random-ized controlled drug trial, the thinking should not be "someone wins" but maybe "I would win without the risks of taking the drug."

I won't even let anyone check my cholesterol, or my prostate-specific antigen (PSA) for that matter. I never submit to screening unless the test is accurate, the disease is important, and something important can be done about it.

TREATING HIGH BLOOD SUGAR

Oral hypoglycemics are prescribed to lower blood sugar in people whose blood sugar qualifies as "type 2 diabetes." All of these drugs lower the blood sugar, or they would not have been licensed. So if I were to treat 100 people, I will lower the blood sugar (or its modern measure, Hemoglobin A1c) to some degree in all 100. The assumption on the part of the FDA was that this must be a good thing to do, an assumption that is widely held by physician and patient alike even today. I say "even today," because the flaw in this reasoning was revealed by three long-term, large trials of lowering the blood sugar of people with type 2 diabetes. Nothing mean-ingful was accomplished; no one was spared a heart attack, renal failure, stroke, amputation, death before their time, or any other of the feared outcomes associated with type 2 diabetes.* For some of the brands of oral hypoglycemics, both newer agents and combinations of older agents, there is an increased incidence of some of these feared outcomes. In forty years of practice, I've never prescribed an oral hypoglycemic drug. I'm waiting for the demonstration of meaningful benefit. I'm waiting for the FDA to demand as much.

It's bad enough that Americans all too often are allowed (encour-aged) to approach medical decisions with a lottery mentality. I under-stand that the citizenries of most states consider playing the state lottery

---

*I presented this argument in the *Clinical Journal of the American Society of Nephrology* 3 (2008): 159–62. This, and the arguments related to primary prevention of heart disease with statins, are developed in detail in *Worried Sick*. One of the counterarguments is that the treat-ment of blood sugar with oral hypoglycemics in these trials was too gentle. That argument is not tenable; the Veterans Affairs Diabetes Trial published the results of treating type 2 dia-betes as aggressively as they could. No benefit resulted (*New England Journal of Medicine* 360 [2009]: 129–39).

a morally defensible exercise. Turning health care into a lottery is morally indefensible.

Small Effectology

There is an "Effectiveness Movement," bloodied and bent but unbowed, that I have championed for fifteen years. We argue that if the intervention has been reasonably well studied and no evidence for meaningful efficacy has been demonstrated, we don't care how well you can do it, or how cheaply, or how efficiently—don't do it!

The forces that thwart the demand for effectiveness are powerful, wealthy, and predictable. Most of the high-ticket items (procedures, tests, and pharmaceuticals) have minimal or no efficacy in RCTs. Yet they are licensed by the FDA. They serve as a food chain for their purveyors at all levels in the process of intervening from manufacturer to regulator and on to insurer and provider. In the case of pharmaceuticals, they are licensed because sufficient efficacy has been demonstrated in a "licensing" RCT to pass muster with the FDA. In the case of devices and procedures, the bar is set much lower, focusing on the safety of the materials rather than the efficacy of their application. Many of these are considered standards of care. They are cash cows for their stakeholders, who may be impervious to a voice such as mine. But I can teach you how to advocate for yourself.

Let's say I have to treat more than fifty people in the hopes of doing something important for one of them—an NNT of >50. Do you believe that's an effective treatment? Nearly all of us involved in biostatistics will tell you that such an outcome is barely measurable and not likely to reproduce. Of the many reasons this is so, several are intrinsic to the design of RCTs in general. One of those, "randomization error," bears emphasis. The first principle of the randomized controlled trial is that subjects are assigned totally randomly to the treated and untreated groups. In this way, all sorts of individual differences can be equally represented in each group: age, gender, weight, what have you. Many of these individual differences can be measured to assure that the distribution is equal. If it is not, there are statistical methods to compensate for identified unequal distributions so that the analysis of outcomes is not biased because of the misdistribution. In the case of unmeasured differences, particularly differences that can't be measured, one has to assume an equal distribution.

Take the example of an RCT of a new drug designed to treat sixty-year-old healthy men for five years to prevent heart attacks. We know that all men age sixty have coronary artery disease, some a little and some a lot, despite being free of symptoms. After randomizing, we assume that the same range of coronary disease is represented in the subjects who will receive the drug and the subjects who will receive a placebo. We might gain reassurance that this is so by doing a coronary catheterization on all the subjects, but that's a procedure that's too invasive and potentially dangerous to be justified for this purpose. We could gain some insight into the distribution of coronary artery disease with less-invasive imaging studies, but these are not sensitive enough for this purpose. So we are forced to assume that the magnitude of coronary artery disease is equal between the treated and untreated groups. What happens if it isn't equal, if it's skewed a bit so that there are a few percent more men with severe disease in one group—say, the untreated control group. It's not terribly unlikely to run into a degree of "skew" this minor. Furthermore, it's not terribly unlikely for the skew to be statistically significant. Statistical significance is defined by computing whether the difference is likely to happen more than five times in a hundred tries; it does not say you know why it happened. In our example, the skew could explain why more in the untreated control group suffered a heart attack and we wouldn't be the wiser. In fact, we'd be inclined to ascribe the difference to the benefit of treatment than to the bias caused by randomization error.

Randomization error is unlikely to cause a major spurious difference in the absolute difference in average outcome. But the likelihood of a small spurious difference causes a scientist such as me to cast a very cautious eye on any scientific paper that is trumpeting small effects. These are the majority of papers in so-called translational research, the studies that are purporting to demonstrate the benefits of plying patients with novel interventions. I term this effort "small effectology" with utter disdain for the fashion in which it has come to dominate clinical thinking and patient decision making. The health of the public would be better served if small effectology was ushered into the archives and the reason for its ignominious demise made transparent. As for the hunt for statistically significant small effects, it is time to cease and desist.

Trolling for Truth in Large Data Sets

There is a variation of the small-effectology theme that deserves wider recognition. The demonstration of efficacy or its lack requires an experiment—an RCT. As we've discussed, RCTs are designed to test efficacy in a reasonable time frame in a highly selected target. Obviously, some hypotheses do not lend themselves to this design. The time frame may be prohibitively long. For example, a hypothesis that a particular intervention in childhood might have a measurable effect in octogenarians is not amenable to study in the lifespan of an investigator. Sometimes, the need to carefully select subjects is limiting because the disease is so rare or so variable in manifestations that no reasonable cohort can be assembled.

These circumstances lead to inventive compromises in design. Some that are commonly employed are so subject to error that no one should take any inference too seriously unless the observation is compelling in magnitude and in specificity, not just in statistical significance. If you look for associations in any large population, you are bound to find many that occur by chance and some that are real associations, but you have no way to know why the associations have occurred. The first point relates to the statistical notion of "significance." One asks whether any association is likely to occur as often by chance and decides that it would not occur by chance more that x times (usually five times) in a 100 ($p < 0.05$). So if you test for associations 100 times, you will find at least the five that occurred by chance.

There are many large data sets, some of which are updated with some frequency. The data are readily available. The urge to test for associations is nearly irresistible. It is at least as great as the likelihood of being fooled by any association that is found. Peter Austin and his colleagues at the University of Toronto provided a sardonic but very telling example in an analysis they published in 2006 ("Testing Multiple Statistical Hypotheses Resulted in Spurious Associations: A Study of Astrological Signs and Health," *Journal of Clinical Epidemiology* 59 [2006]: 964–69). They had access to all sorts of health data on over 10 million residents of Ontario. They performed an analysis asking whether any of the 223 of the most common reasons for hospitalization associated with a person's astrologic sign. They found several reproducible statistical associations, such as between being born a Sagittarian and fracturing one's arm, or being born under Leo and suffering a gastrointestinal hemorrhage. If they corrected mathematically for the number of tests required to tease out such associations, none remained. But the lessons remain: no one should pummel large data sets seeking insights for which they were not designed in the first place without a great deal of trepidation, and no one should place stock in any inferences drawn from such exercises without even more trepidation.

That's why one year, butter is bad for you, and the next, margarine is bad for you. Pshaw.

The "Absence of Proof Is Not Proof of Absence" Muddle

As I said above, for me to consider a health effect important, I need to see an NNT smaller than 20. I'm pretty hard-nosed about that since I am convinced that the hazard of unnecessary, ineffective treatments greatly outweighs the possibility of withholding interventions that advantage many only a little or very few a lot. However, the consensus among those who understand and study these considerations is more liberal; most would acquiesce to an NNT less than 50. Here's a partial list of treatments that would not even qualify at this level of effectiveness based on RCTs designed to test their efficacy:

- Coronary artery bypass grafts, angioplasties, or stents to save lives, strengthen the heart, or improve symptoms
- Arthroscopy for knee pain
- Any surgery for backache
- Statin therapy to reduce cholesterol and thereby save lives
- Oral hypoglycemics to prevent the ravages of type 2 diabetes
- Newer antidepressants for situational depression
- Drugs for decreased bone density
- PSA screening and radical prostatectomy to save lives
- Screening mammography to save lives
- Many a cancer treatment to save lives

The list of treatments that have been studied and fail to meet the NNT <50 criterion goes on and on, including many of the new drugs touted as "breakthroughs." Many surgical treatments have yet to be studied. From my perspective as a clinician who has cared for patients and taught students for over four decades, if I have to treat more than twenty patients to do something really meaningful for one, the treatment is marginal; I do not prescribe or advocate it and would have no problem if it was not covered by health insurance. Furthermore, designing trials to test whether new or old treatments meet this one-in-twenty level of efficacy is not difficult, expensive, or time-consuming. We could look at a future when we would no longer be marketed to prescribe and consume minimally effective treatments, or treatments that offered no important improvement compared to those that are older and tried-and-true. And using the methodology of CER, we can use the data on efficacious interventions to assault the contemporary pharmacopoeia and weed out the ineffective in common use.

Reducing Risks

I take pains to express efficacy in absolute terms, although I've been selective in my vocabulary in this regard, emphasizing NNTs because this metric tends not to cause unfounded optimism. For example, imagine a sudden-onset dramatic illness from which 96 percent of patients recover to live at least another five years. I undertake an RCT of a drug and learn that 98 percent on that drug live at least another five years. That's an absolute reduction in mortality of 2 percent, which in this hypothetical study (given the number of subjects) is statistically significant. Since we're talking about a sudden-onset dramatic illness, it is unreasonable to ask an acutely ill patient to ponder the value of a 2 percent absolute reduction in risk of death in five years. Such a discussion needs to play out dispassionately before one becomes ill. A 2 percent absolute reduction in five-year mortality is essentially equivalent to an NNT of 50, or on the cusp. If fifty patients take the pill every day for five years, it is likely that only one wasn't wasting his or her time. It is certainly not mandatory that one take the pill every day for the next five years for such marginal efficacy. But before discounting the treatment in light of NNT, perhaps there is ancillary information that might turn you into a pill taker. What does the pill cost in terms of potential adverse effects, if not out-of-pocket expenditure?

However, there is another way to express the efficacy of this drug. Mortality dropped from 4 percent to 2 percent, an absolute difference of 2 percent. But the drop from 4 percent to 2 percent is also a relative decrease in mortality of 50 percent. If I offered you a pill that dropped your five-year mortality 50 percent, you'd likely leap at it and be far more tolerant of its costliness. Most would. Most would envision themselves dead without the drug and attaining a 50 percent chance of living with it. Our reflexive tendency to magnify the implication of relative frequencies has not escaped marketing agendas or, for that matter, the agendas of the research scientists who are likely to strut with such an "important" result.

Every clinical investigator and medical-journal editor worth his or her salt is aware of our proclivity to grasp at relative risk reductions and similar ways to express outcome data. Yet relative-frequency calculations are likely to be featured in the abstract of the paper and in the introductory statement that many (most) read without reading further. They are likely to find their way into the media and the marketing with great frequency. The clinical journals and the FDA seem comfortable looking the other way at this practice. Of course, one can find the absolute frequencies (the

96 percent and 98 percent) and the difference in absolute frequencies (2 percent) in the body of the paper. Sometimes there's even an NNT. But nowhere will you find a bold proclamation that you must know the absolute frequencies before you can interpret relative risk reduction. Clearly, this represents an attempt to sway the thinking of the audience toward the prejudicial thinking of the proponents. Such is a shameful denigration of one of the ethical foundations of clinical research: equipoise.

In 1987 Benjamin Freedman, an ethicist at McGill University, published an essay in the *New England Journal of Medicine* titled "Equipoise and the Ethics of Clinical Research." Freedman defined equipoise as "a state of genuine uncertainty on the part of the clinical investigator regarding the comparative therapeutic merits of each arm." Others have echoed this sentiment over the years, and some try to take it to heart. Equipoise in clinical research is the lofty goal to which everyone should aspire. Having performed RCTs at the National Institutes of Health early in my career, I can tell you that it is possible to design a trial adhering to the principle of equipoise, and it is possible to analyze the data adhering to the principle of equipoise, but it is difficult to recruit patients into a trial unless you have a hope that you will be offering them an advantage. If you think the experimental intervention is worthless, how can you undertake recruitment?

I can tolerate violating equipoise only to this degree. It is unconscionable to violate it in design, data analysis, or presentation of results. But violating in all three of these aspects has become the rule, particularly in industry-sponsored trials. Therefore, to my way of thinking, RCTs should no longer be the purview of industry, nor should the FDA's process of "New Drug Applications" have any taint of prejudice toward the sponsors. Currently, the FDA is dependent on application fees from sponsors to supplement its federal budget and is both allowed and inclined to include many an adviser who has industry ties. Furthermore, clinical journals, the clinical audience, and the FDA should not countenance language designed to distort the clinical decision-making process. It is possible to turn these principles into regulations. We will examine such reforms in a later chapter.

By the way, the hypothetical acute illness we've just discussed is not at all hypothetical. Today, the frequency that well men live for five years from their first heart attack is about 96 percent. Survival frequency increases to 98 percent by taking a baby aspirin daily. That may be a marginal NNT, but for a baby aspirin, I'd go for it.

Heart of My Heart

I ended chapter 1 with the Crestor canard to reemphasize the major points I had been making about medical shills. I'll close this chapter with a discussion of coronary artery bypass graft surgery (CABG) to reemphasize the consequences of making medical decisions based on flawed information. CABGs were the product of a very exciting time in medicine and surgery. It was the 1960s. Major advances in anesthesiology and in the postoperative care of patients allowed surgeons to undertake procedures in very ill patients without killing them. This unleashed a wave of surgical innovation, including in cardiac surgery. For the first time, patients facing death from diseases that severely damage heart valves could be taken to surgery and recover with a functioning new heart valve. These procedures, now fine-tuned, remain miraculous to this day.

Meanwhile, there were great advances in our understanding of angina and heart attacks. Both reflect limitations in the flow of blood to portions of the heart muscle. "Hardening of the arteries" is the buildup of concretions in the major arteries of the heart. The concretions are termed plaque, and the process is termed atherosclerosis or coronary artery disease. It is apparent in autopsies and also apparent in life if one performs X-rays having injected particular dyes directly into the coronary arteries. The procedure is termed cardiac catheterization, and the resulting image is a coronary angiogram. It was posited that these growing plaques were slowly narrowing the arteries, resulting in angina and heart attacks. It makes sense, doesn't it?

It surely made sense to the skilled cadre of heart surgeons who leaped at a technical solution. Why not devise a conduit that carries blood around the occlusion—a coronary artery bypass? They perfected their techniques in the laboratory, usually using dogs. To this day, there is no regulatory barrier against taking a surgical technique from the laboratory to the operating room. There is peer review, but the peerage was enamored with the technological achievement.

The rest is history. Well over 500,000 CABGs are performed in the United States each year on patients of all ages with coronary artery disease, including the elderly. Between 2 percent and 8 percent of these patients die without ever leaving the hospital following the surgery. About half have a difficult recovery over the first six months. About a third are still suffering measurable memory loss at one year as a consequence of their CABG. But all survivors, their families, and their greater communities applaud their courage and are convinced that their life has been spared. Celebrities trumpet triumph, and everyone knows their bypass count. "I had a quintuple . . ."

From the very beginning of the planting of the CABG patch, there was controversy. Were these survivors advantaged by the miracle or just lucky to survive the CABG? Through the 1970s and well into the 1980s, the CABG enterprise thrived, particularly in the United States, and came to consume a major portion of the "health-care dollar." In so doing, it nurtured the income and the egos of heart surgeons and their supporting players and, to an even greater degree, spawned the current colossal American hospital center. Still, there were those who doubted, including those who represented the pioneers of evidence-based medicine and the use of the RCT. The result was three randomized controlled trials of men with angina who were treated with a CABG or with the standard of medical therapy in the 1970s and 1980s. Two of the trials were American—one sponsored by the Veterans Administration, the other by the National Institutes of Health—and one was European. Many hundreds of men volunteered, were randomized, and were followed for many years—for over a decade in the case of the European trial. The primary outcome to be assessed was survival. The primary finding is that CABG did not improve survival in any of the trials compared to medical therapy.

Talk about equipoise. The number of stakeholders who balked at this result was legion. Fortunately for them, there was a light in their bloated tunnel. There is one subset that is obviously advantaged by CABG, a subset that shone through the haze and has since proven a durable candidate for the procedure. This subset has a particular distribution of plaque among the two major coronary arteries, one to the right side of the heart and the other to the left. The one to the left is the left main artery, which shortly branches into two vessels. Patients with angina and occluding plaque concentrated in the left main artery have a 65 percent five-year survival on medical therapy and an 85 percent five-year survival if they survive CABG. That's a 20 percent absolute difference in survival—an NNT of 5! But . . . only about 3 percent of patients with angina have isolated left main disease. That means you would have to do a cardiac catheterization with coronary angiography on 100 patients to find the three with left main disease. That procedure carries a much higher percentage of serious adverse events, including a 1 to 2 percent fatality rate. Left main disease offered up the glimmer of hope the CABG enterprise desperately wanted, but it is far from a home run.

Again: talk about equipoise. Given the left main result, the investigators involved in these trials returned to the data to test alternative hypotheses. Was the result more encouraging if another single vessel was involved, or any combination of the right coronary artery and the two branches of the left main? This was one of the aforementioned secondary analyses that serve no more than to generate hypotheses. That it was an exploratory analysis was barely acknowledged; data were mined to come up with a statistically significant minor survival advantage if all three major vessels were bypassed, particularly if the patient already had a weak heart muscle. Exploratory analysis was damned. This was truth. Furthermore, it is hard to imagine that the notion of bypassing occlusions is faulty given the success with left main disease and now the putative success with three-vessel disease. It was open season on any occlusion that could be bypassed, and it remains so to this day. One of my favorite and most respected heart surgeons once said to me that doubts vanish when the bypass is completed and he holds a pink heart beating in his hands.

Now you know the science that underpins the millions of bypasses that have been perpetrated on millions of Americans and fewer but still impressive numbers of others in resource-advantaged countries. It is consummate sophistry.

The doubting is no match for the power of the CABG enterprise. The result of the STICH trial was published in the *New England Journal of Medicine* in 2011. This was a multicenter trial recruiting 1,212 patients between 2002 and 2007, all with coronary artery disease resulting in weakening of the heart muscle and heart failure. All received the best medical therapy could offer. Half were randomized to CABG. Those that survived the surgery enjoyed absolutely no survival advantage over those spared the knife. Do you think this will diminish the enthusiasm of the CABG enterprise?

My favorite George Bernard Shaw quote comes from the author's preface to *The Doctor's Dilemma*:

> It may also be necessary to hang a man or pull down a house. But we take good care not to make the hangman and the housebreaker the judges of that. If we did, no man's neck would be safe and no man's house stable.

4

If We Build It, They Will Come

THE PROCEDURES AND DEVICES GAMBIT

In this book, I am arming all of us, the Citizen Patients, with the knowledge to demand a health-care system that cannot sell us a pig in a poke, let alone profit from doing so. Americans are enamored of anything that's new and shiny, particularly if it is "high-tech" and expensive. There are many examples where this fixation has led to progress for some if not all. The Apple Corporation is a case in point. EMI, the British music recording company, turned its attention from recording the Beatles to medical imaging, and now we consider CT scans as ordinary as we once considered routine X-rays. But there are many examples where the newest and shiniest turned out to be useless or a lemon. Such do not survive long in a free market, as the American automobile industry found out.

In the medical world, however, consumerism is gravely compromised. "Caveat emptor" seems irrelevant if something is already indemnified by one's health-insurance policy. Patients seldom view themselves as consumers. Patients, by definition, are ill and seldom inclined to comparison shop, and even more seldom do they view themselves as purchasing items with which they are familiar from prior purchases. Patients are inherently patsies who depend on the sales pitch of the various providers.

Arming patients with knowledge is a piecemeal solution to the imbalance between an individual patient and a particular provider in the clinical arena. In chapter 3, we considered how an agency such as the FDA is charged with providing security when it comes to pharmaceuticals—and how well this mandate is served. In this chapter, we will consider whether society has constructed adequate safeguards for another aspect of the provision of health care: procedures, devices, and other widgets. There is a heated debate regarding the traditional regulatory approach to doing things to patients and putting things in patients. It has long been argued that as long as the "things" were not inherently toxic, no regulatory oversight is needed because efficacy is more dependent on procedural competence than the procedure itself. The Citizen Patient needs to understand this debate and weigh in—there is much at stake.

Fortunately, the Citizen Patient is not alone in coming to grips with a need to assure that medical interventions offer benefits that are scientifically validated. But the ally in this endeavor is not the regulators or the legislators; sadly, these resources are wallowing in preconceptions that are whipped by stakeholders. It is the judiciary that is stepping up to the plate.

A Stent for Daubert

In 1993 the U.S. Supreme Court issued its decision in *Daubert v. Merrell Dow Pharmaceuticals, Inc.* (509 U.S. 579, 584–87). The case was a product-liability suit brought by the Daubert family and other plaintiffs against Merrell Dow regarding the drug bendectin. This drug is effective in suppressing the nausea that can plague the first trimester of pregnancy. Unfortunately, Mrs. Daubert and the other plaintiffs who were exposed to this drug bore children with phocomelia, a fetal growth defect leading to short limbs. This harkened to the tragedy associated with thalidomide exposures that led to the Estes-Kefauver amendment to the law regulating the FDA thirty years earlier—the amendment that called for the FDA to assess efficacy and license drugs based on their benefit-risk profile. Given the thalidomide precedent, the plaintiffs and their attorneys argued that bendectin is similarly toxic to fetal development.

A case like this works its way up through lower courts to arrive at the U.S. Supreme Court. At each stage, experts for the plaintiffs argued guilt by association given the thalidomide precedent. Experts for the defense argued that phocomelia was an exceedingly rare birth defect—and no less rare if exposure to bendectin is involved. The Supreme Court was asked to offer some solution to the battle of the experts. That solution is known as the Daubert Standard or Daubert Rule and pertains to federal jurisdictions. About half the states have adopted it as well.

According to the Daubert Standard of Expert Opinion, no longer should scientific information influence courts, judges, or juries simply because an expert presenting the information has the credentials and hubris to declare it "generally accepted." Rather, judges have a "gatekeeping" responsibility. To serve that responsibility, they are to assure the "relevance" and the "reliability" of the scientific basis of the opinion any expert is tendering. The case was remanded to the U.S. Court of Appeals for the Ninth Circuit, where the opinion written by Chief Judge Alex Kozinski took advantage of principles of evidence-based medicine to hone the notions of "relevance" and "reliability." (These principles of evidence-based medicine are the theme of chapter 3.) The most weight is to be given to the results of experiments, randomized controlled trials (RCTs) in particular, and the least weight given to statements of consensus and personal opinion. The Daubert Standard is implemented when one of the parties in a trial—the judge or the attorneys for either the plaintiff or the defense—makes a pretrial motion that particular expert testimony should not be presented to the jury because it lacks "relevance" or "reliability." A separate trial follows that puts the science to the test of the Daubert Standard. The judge is to decide whether the evidence is of sufficient "relevance" and "reliability" to be presented to a jury. If not, the case goes no further in that jurisdiction.

As is clear from the substance of this book and my previous writings, I have a career-long fascination with the way "science," particularly clinical science, influences socially constructed truths—that is, belief systems and the common sense. I was delighted twenty years ago by the Daubert opinion. I have written about its implications, starting with a paper titled "A Keyboard for Daubert" published in the *Journal of Occupational and Environmental Medicine* in 1996. I have lectured about it at law schools and elsewhere from my perspective as a clinical investigator. There is no doubt that the Daubert Standard has rendered science more transparent in the legal context and that this transparency has spilled over into many aspects of society. However, neither I nor other commentators are convinced the Daubert Rule has often advantaged a jury by excluding scientifically unsound information. After all, most suits are brought when the science leaves room for uncertainty. If the conclusion is considered incontrovertible, there would be either no need for a Daubert hearing or for the suit in the first place. The occasional judge is willing to assume responsibility for overlooking minor degrees of uncertainty in finding the science irrelevant or unreliable. But most are unwilling to take such a leap, in which case the judge will let the jury decide on the "reliability" of the science by employing whatever wisdom a "jury of peers" can mobilize.

As an aside, I have long pleaded with my colleagues who are legal scholars, including one who was a member of the committee responsible for writing and updating the Federal Rules of Evidence, to stop using the word "reliable" in this context. In science, reliability speaks to whether one gets the same result every time one does any particular assessment. "Validity" is the scientific term that speaks to whether your assessment or its interpretation actually does what you designed it to do. In science, you can get the same spurious result every time if the same biases are operating. In that circumstance, the science is reliable but not valid. If validity were substituted for reliability in Rule 702, which defines the Daubert Standard, there would be a bit less dissonance between science and the law in the courtroom and far less in scholarly writings.

Chief Justice William Rehnquist dissented on part of the Daubert decision. He raised this concern: "I do not doubt that Rule 702 confides to the judge some gatekeeping responsibility in deciding questions of the admissibility of proffered expert testimony. But I do not think [509 US 601] it imposes on them either the obligation or the authority to become amateur scientists in order to perform that role." As one wag put it: "Judges have enough trouble putting on their robes. Now you want them to do statistics." After all, the traditional model of a judge is as a wise but empty vessel into which one pours all the facts and then shakes, and the blend that pours out is truth. But if the facts are a great number of data points, blending requires analytic skills that must first be learned. That is rendered all the more difficult because the data points are likely to be couched in language that is foreign to all but certain aficionados. Imagine what it must be like to hear the evidence in something like a patent-infringement suit brought against one of the software giants.

One solution is to render the Daubert hearing didactic and interactive to take advantage of judges who are particularly quick students willing to question presenting experts. I have been involved as a presenting expert in several such hearings (relating to my research on workplace health and safety). Sometimes, this is a satisfying educational experience for both the presenting expert and the judge; sometimes it is not. Because of these challenges, about half the states have created "science courts." Usually, highly respected senior state judges are recruited to the task of serving as "finders of fact" in technologically demanding cases that come before the science court. There is also the Advanced Science and Technology

Adjudication Resource (ASTAR) Program, a congressionally mandated continuing-education program designed to enhance the analytic skills of the science judges. The judges are freed up from their dockets to participate for several days in intensive seminars on particularly relevant technological topics. The programs are usually held on university campuses and hosted by the supreme court of that state. One of the ASTAR themes is euphemistically called the "Judges' Medical School." Usually 100 to 150 judges interact with a small, carefully chosen faculty. I have been privileged to serve on several of these faculties, and I consider the experience to be the pinnacle for an educator. It's a give-and-take between highly trained and experienced scholarly intellects that are looking at the same issues from very different perspectives.

At one of the Judges' Medical Schools, we constructed a mock Daubert hearing. My role was as the expert for the plaintiff. At issue was whether my testimony should be admitted. The "judge" was the assembly of state judges in attendance. Here's the case, titled "Death by Angioplasty":

William Jones is a 56-year-old well-known and well-liked successful businessman who is highly respected in the community. His lifestyle includes a daily morning jog. He was jogging along comfortably one morning when he noted a squeezing sensation in the middle of his chest. He tried to ignore it but it grew in intensity, with the pain radiating toward his left shoulder. He was stopped in his tracks, sweating, anxious, and scared. The pain subsided pretty rapidly once he stopped but recurred as soon as he commenced walking, this time toward home. He stopped again, sat down on the curb and called his wife on his cell phone. When she arrived, he felt himself except somewhat foolish and was willing to walk home. She would have none of that and took him to their family internist, Dr. Howell. Dr. Howell listened to the experience and said that this could be little else than angina. Dr. Howell had a treadmill in his office and asked Bill to try it out. Before long, the pain recurred, and there were changes on the cardiogram suggesting inadequate blood supply to the heart. Bill was ushered to a neighboring office, the office of Dr. Clayton, the cardiologist. Dr. Clayton concurred with Dr. Howell. He told Bill and his wife that it was advisable he undergo a coronary angiogram with a view toward identifying any correctable occlusive plaques in his heart. If the plaques were amenable to angioplasty, Dr. Clayton would perform that at the time of the study. If not, he would refer Bill to a heart surgeon for bypass surgery (CABG).

There followed a lengthy explanation of the procedure and its potential for harm. Angioplasty involved placing a catheter with a balloon at the tip into the center of the plaque and blowing up the balloon. That would fracture the plaque and open up the vessel. If feasible, a stent would be inserted to keep the blood vessel open and allow blood to flow freely to the heart muscle. A stent is a metal conduit, in this case one that is coated with chemicals to prevent blood clots. Bill was asked to sign a permission slip that stated he understood the procedure and its potential for complications. Potential complications include rupture of the vessel, heart attack, and death. Bill underwent catheterization that afternoon. Sadly, he suffered all three major complications. He didn't die in the catheterization laboratory; he was rushed to the operating room, where heart surgeons tried to bypass the grief. It's a horrible outcome but it occurs in 1 to 2 percent of patients like Bill.

Much to Dr. Howell's surprise, Mrs. Jones brings suit against him. The complaint was that the permission slip was inadequate if not fraudulent. It explained the procedure and the potential risks but never in the process of giving his permission was Mr. Jones informed that this procedure wouldn't advantage him in the least. It would not increase the likelihood of escaping symptomatic or damaging heart disease. It was worthless. Mr. Jones was hardly fully informed when he acquiesced to having the procedure.

The suit could not be brought against the manufacturer of the stent for reasons we will discuss shortly, but mainly such suits are thwarted by a U.S. Supreme Court decision that provides manufacturers with tort immunity as soon as their widget is sanctioned by the FDA. A standard malpractice suit could not be brought against Dr. Howell either. His practice was up to the standards of his community. But if the science supports Mrs. Jones's contention, Dr. Howell is indeed guilty of a form of malpractice. The mock Daubert hearing was requested by the attorneys for the defense, who argued that I was not a qualified expert and therefore my testimony should not be admitted to the trial proceedings. It is true that I'm not a cardiologist. I did spend five years as an Established Investigator of the American Heart Association, which bolstered my extensive credentials as someone capable of a critical analysis of the evidentiary basis for coronary angiography. My playacting attorney, the attorney for Mrs. Jones, argued that it was the science that was critical and that I was perfectly competent to present the science, cardiologist or not. I went on to explain that science to the assembly of judges. Our focus was coronary angioplasty with or without stenting.

I knew that arguing Mrs. Jones's case before the assembled judges was an uphill battle against their collective preconceptions. The five-year mortality for a well man after his first heart attack has dropped from 50 percent to 5 percent in one generation. The line of people who are taking credit for this happy turn of events is very long. At the head of the line stand the cardiovascular surgeons and interventional cardiologists. They bask in the praise of the media and of their celebrity patients who consider them saviors. If you have survived one of these modern medical miracles unscathed, you feel blessed to live in such a medically advantaged community. If symptoms return, it seems so reasonable to return to this technological fountain. If you survived scathed, or if you succumbed, it means that even modern medical miracles were no match for the magnitude of your affliction. This is the social construction that every American has been taught and nearly every American has accepted. I looked at the assemblage of judges and noticed a lot of gray hair. In America, you can assume such an audience is replete with survivors, or at least with people who have a loved one who is a survivor. I have been decrying this sophistry in lectures and in print throughout all the decades it took for it to become common wisdom. There is no doubt in my mind that interventional cardiology has written the bleakest chapter in the entire history of Western medicine, second only to that written about cardiovascular surgery for coronary artery disease. Today, I am bolstered by an informative science, which I explained to the judges.

I started out on my crusade by relying on first principles, but as technology evolved, so did the clinical science refuting the efficacy of the angioplasty enterprise. Coronary angioplasty was the brainchild of German cardiologist Andreas Gruentzig over two decades ago. One has to wonder how he managed to convince peers, let alone patients, that it was a good idea to stick a balloon into a plaque in a major coronary artery, blow the balloon up, and burst the plaque asunder. We now know that a significant percentage of these patients suffer an acute heart attack. Furthermore, when this trick is applied to occlusions of the arteries to the head, strokes result more often than not. But it was 1977, and medicine was enamored with technological progress. Furthermore, there were no Institutional Review Boards, regulatory agencies, or other ethical barriers to be breeched before one's heartfelt "good idea" could arrive at the bedside. When it comes to surgical techniques, there are no such hurdles today. The surgeon is only accountable to conscience, peers, and issues in reimbursement. In comparison, if I go into my laboratory and concoct a pill that I believe will help my patients with rheumatoid arthritis and convince them to give it a try without leaping through all kinds of regulatory and ethical barriers, I risk losing my license, my admitting privileges, and much more.

As I said, it was 1977, and the CABG industry was revving into full swing. The only piece of the action that still remained the purview of cardiologists was diagnosis, including coronary angiography. The glory and the gold went to the surgeons. Gruentzig offered the cardiology world the promise of leveling the playing field, and they leaped at it. Before long, Americans in particular were lying still for angioplasty as often as for CABGS, and the frequency of both skyrocketed, so that instead of just 500,000 CABGS per year, both CABGS and angioplasties approached 1 million per year each. There was a rich science comparing the results of the two approaches. Outcomes are comparable, as are costs, though angioplasty is a far-less-brutal procedure. Since it was accepted that CABGS are terrific, it was assumed that since angioplasty was as good, it was terrific also. I wrote that since the data for any benefit from CABG was so marginal, the syllogism would hold that angioplasty was worthless too. No one listened.

Everyone's ears pricked up when it was shown that both bypass grafts and arteries that had been subjected to angioplasty have a very great propensity to clot off and occlude again in the near term. Enter the era of the stent. Several types of bare metal stents were developed and studied in RCTs comparing angioplasty with and without stenting. These studies were not just seed trials; they were required by the FDA to exclude toxicity from the materials used to construct the stent. These stents were no more harmful than doing angioplasty without stenting. They also were no more efficacious in preventing fatal or nonfatal heart attacks. They also clotted off again and as quickly. This last observation has unleashed great technological innovations. Scientists are looking for ways to coat the stent so it won't occlude as quickly. In recent years, they have made a great deal of progress in this regard. Much to the consternation of these scientists and all the other stakeholders, they have found to their horror in efficacy trials that these coated stents may not clot but seem to increase the likelihood of heart attacks six months after the procedure when compared to angioplasty without stenting or angioplasty with bare metal stents. Of course, rather than give up the ghost, the enterprise calls for prescribing clopidigrel (an agent that interferes with the clotting mechanism) as a theoretical solution to the harm they were causing with their newfangled gizmos.

After all the hundreds of trials comparing different versions of angioplasty one to the other and different versions of angioplasty to different versions of CABG, science turned to the meat of the matter. Was any of this violence to coronary arteries doing more for the patient than the best of medical therapy—a few pills and some advice about getting on with life? The answer resounds in the negative. No patient is rewarded in terms of longevity, incidence of heart attacks, or likelihood of chest pain for having submitted to these expensive technical and technological feats, and many suffer harm in the course of the procedure. Here are my picks as the best of the lot of RCTs comparing violence with perspective:

- In the RITA-2 trial, 1,000 carefully selected patients with angina in 1997 were randomized to angioplasty or medical therapy. The consequences were last reported in 2003. Those initially randomized to noninvasive treatment did as well as those who underwent angioplasty.
- Matthias Pfisterer and his Swiss coinvestigators randomized elderly patients with angina to optimized medical therapy or early invasive therapy with angioplasty (with or without stenting) or to bypass graft surgery and followed them for four years. There was no advantage to the early invasive strategy in terms of death or myocardial infarction (MI).
- The COURAGE trial is particularly damning: no one with stable angina should be told that angioplasty, with or without stenting, prevents a heart attack or stroke or prolongs life.
- In the multicenter OAT trial funded by the National Institutes of Health, 2,000 patients were recruited within a month of their heart attack because they had persistent blockage of the relevant coronary artery and heart damage. All received optimal medical care; half were randomized to also undergo angioplasty and stent placement. Over the next four years, there was no difference between the two groups in terms of recurrent heart attack, death, or heart failure. If anything, those with the stents fared less well.
- In BARI-2D, the comparison was with high-risk patients with stable angina and type 2 diabetes. Over 2,000 were randomized. There is no advantage to prompt revascularization over medical therapy for coronary artery disease in this setting.
- The MASS-II trial randomized 611 patients with multivessel

coronary artery disease and stable angina with preserved heart muscle function. At one year, there was no difference in cardiac death or acute MI between patients in the CABG, angioplasty, or medical-therapy groups.

There you have it. The leading state "science" judges in the audience were dumbfounded. The chief justice of the host state and several other justices were dumbfounded. The judge who was role-playing the defense attorney for Dr. Clayton's malpractice insurance company was silenced. The judge who was role-playing as the plaintiff's attorney on behalf of Mrs. Jones smiled. The assembled judges were asked to vote on whether, according to the Daubert Standard, my testimony should be allowed before the jury. They voted overwhelmingly in the affirmative.

So why is it that over a million such invasive procedures are performed in the United States each year and indemnified by all private insurers, by Medicaid programs, and by Medicare? If angioplasty was a pharmaceutical, do you think the FDA could find a way to license it when the critical data prerequisite to licensing it was a series of negative randomized controlled trials? But procedures are not subjected to licensing, and devices such as stents are held to a much lower standard; they must be safe in the short term, but there need not be a demonstration of efficacy. But the drug-eluting stents led to more harm in some studies. Shouldn't the FDA remove them from the market? The FDA convened an advisory committee, on which stakeholders were well represented, and came to the conclusion that prescribing clopidigrel for these stented patients was safety enough. Hence, the FDA is not standing between Americans and the invasive cardiology and cardiovascular surgery community. Since the coronary artery plaque-removal enterprise is the recipient of a sizable portion of the "health-care dollar," it has the fiscal wherewithal to make certain that it is favored in the media, in Congress, and generally in the mind of the public. A few of the leading medical journalists, such as John Carey in *Business Week*, have had the editorial support to display the relevant science as early as 2005, but such efforts are overwhelmed by the miasma of marketing.

How about the doctors who do this violence to our coronary arteries? Some have bent their moral compass to an unconscionable if not illegal degree. Atul Gawande displayed an example of such in a brilliant essay, "The Cost Conundrum" (*New Yorker*, December 6, 2010). Most are not misanthropes. The "thought leaders" are well aware of the science. But most can overcome my kind of compunctions with three rationales.

One rationale I call the "folly of peer review." These interventional cardiologists and cardiovascular surgeons are prominent in their communities, where their incomes, if nothing else, command respect. It is human nature for such people to come together bursting with pride that "my stent is bigger than your stent." It is not human nature to applaud the "peer" who questions whether the stenting should have been done in the first place. The folly of peer review is not exclusive to my guild; it operates widely, including on Wall Street when wizards were bundling bigger junk mortgages.

Another rationale is science based. All RCTs specify the population that is recruited, including criteria such as age, coincidental diseases, prior cardiac history, current symptoms, and the like. It is easy for an interventionalist to tell a patient that he or she is different from the subjects in the studies and that, "In my experience, this works for patients like you." For all I know, the interventionalist is correct—but believing so is a matter of faith in the face of the precedent that medical therapy works better in all other circumstances. For me, creating a theory that is self-serving is the essence of quackery. Any such theory should be subjected to testing before it can or should be offered based "on my experience."

If you go to an American emergency room with chest pain, everything will be done to get you to the cardiac catheterization laboratory as quickly as possible and on to angioplasty (with or without stent) or bypass grafting if the eyes of the beholding interventionalist are convinced it's feasible. They are in such a hurry because it's so difficult to demonstrate that you are better off for the procedure(s) if there is any delay. Since it is believed that the procedures are inherently sensible, it follows that they should be done as quickly as possible, with little if any time to make an informed medical decision. This race from the door to the catheterization suite is lucrative for the hospital, but it is driven by metaphysics and not by data. In some studies, you are better off if your local hospital lacks a cardiac catheterization laboratory, thus sparing you from this vortex. Cardiologists are wont to point to data from Denmark and elsewhere that suggests that those who are transferred most rapidly from a community hospital to a hospital with a catheterization laboratory are better off in the long run. Of course, those who are transferred most rapidly are the least sick, or they couldn't be transferred so rapidly. No patient is able to question the "door to balloon" credo when experiencing chest pain; pain, anxiety, and fear blunt his or her critical capacities, as well as those of a loved one. Certainly, any patient would be better off if the options had been explored beforehand and preferences established. However, that is another example of a piecemeal approach to informed medical decision making. The Citizen Patient needs to demand that these options be explored in an accessible and transparent fashion. Would anyone agree to a rapid transfer to the cardiac catheterization laboratory in the emergency room if the cardiologist admitted that scientists have tried and failed to show you have anything to gain?

Speaking of scientific testing, I find it striking that interventional cardiology and cardiovascular surgery offers no advantage over medical therapy in terms of symptoms for all the many clinical subsets that have been studied. As we'll discuss in chapter 6, far-less-dramatic "interventions" tend to have an enormous placebo effect if the providers exude enthusiasm, the recipients arrive with preconceptions of benefit, and the result is colored by the need for justification by both parties. I would have thought that the only way to test the efficacy of interventional procedures for chest pain was by randomizing volunteers to the procedure or to a sham procedure. A sham-surgery trial was done many years ago for an early version of coronary artery bypass surgery for severe angina with a negative result; all patients were anaesthetized and all had a skin incision, but only half had the actual bypass performed. The likelihood of improvement was the same whether or not the bypass was performed. In all the trials listed above, despite placebo bias, invasiveness does no better than medical therapy in saving lives or sparing heart attacks for every form of coronary artery disease that has been studied. I will assume that holds for every form of coronary artery disease that has yet to be studied until a well-designed RCT convinces me otherwise.

The FDA and Devices

As I said, there is no regulatory precedent regarding surgical techniques. Surgeons gain fame and glory for inventing new techniques that other surgeons respect. There is also a long history of surgeons inventing surgical instruments, scissors or clamps or the like, that are then patented and purveyed as a "What's His Name" Widget, such as a Kelly Clamp. Sometimes these represent fluff; sometimes they are technical advances that advantage patients by enhancing surgical skillfulness or efficiency. Take the example of all the surgery that can be done in various body cavities by inserting specially designed surgical instruments through small wounds and directing their action by observation through a fiberoptic scope inserted through another small wound. Lots of things can be done to diseases in the abdomen, pelvis, and joints by such methodology with vastly shortened recovery. All this evolved with the most gentle of regulatory oversight. Even devices that are left in the body are still only lightly regulated.

Prior to 1976, a laissez-faire attitude toward surgical instruments and techniques was applied to devices that could be left on or in the patient. The notion was that a device differs from a pharmaceutical because no chemical is dissolving. In the early 1970s, there was a spate of failed cardiac pacemakers and of complications from the Dalkon Shield intrauterine contraceptive device. In 1976, after several years of congressional debate and discussion, President Gerald R. Ford signed into law the Medical Device Amendments to the Food, Drug, and Cosmetic Act. The amendments classified devices according to their hazardous nature so that the amount of oversight could be appropriately graduated. Class I devices required no new oversight; tongue depressors, bandages, and the like had to meet manufacturing standards and "good manufacturing practice" (GMP) regulations, but little else. Class II devices were wheelchairs, impact-resistant lenses, and the like that had to meet performance standards in addition to GMP. Class III devices were those that involved invading the body and had obvious potential for harm. Class III devices require FDA premarket approval. Most in Class III that make it to the market garnered approval through the "510(k) clearance pathway," which stipulates merely that the device is "substantially equivalent" to a device already on the market.

If not deemed "substantially equivalent," the standard for approval that pertains to pharmaceuticals did not seem appropriate for devices and other "things." In addition to the distinction drawn with pharmaceuticals in terms of their biochemistry (devices are not absorbed into the body chemistry), it was argued that the safety of devices depends largely on their being used properly. The risk/benefit ratio of a lens implanted in the eye to replace a cataract or of an anesthesia machine or glucose monitor is as much a function of its proper usage as it materials and engineering. Therefore, the FDA is willing to accept observational studies rather than require the deductive gold standard for pharmaceuticals: the RCT. Furthermore, the FDA felt some obligation to educate practitioners and patients about the safe use of devices and to exercise authority to notify and ban usage in the case of deception or risk of injury. This line of reasoning lowers the threshold for licensing devices well below that of pharmaceuticals.

The FDA's Center for Devices and Radiologic Health is revisiting the fashion in which the 510(k) clearance pathway is administered. Most of the effort is aimed at making the process more predictable and therefore more efficient. There is a great deal of pressure on the FDA not to stifle innovation. The dialectic is not straightforward. "Innovation" is an American calling card; we make novel things and thereby create industries and jobs. But the devices to be regulated by the 510(k) clearance pathway are not your usual novel things. The market cannot be counted on to reject the latest golly-gee-whiz widget because it's too costly, unreliable, or useless. The judgment that a new device is "substantially equivalent" cannot be assumed on face value; it must be tested. We've been burned too often—for example, when we learn from lawsuits that a novel state-of-the-art hip replacement wears out sooner than the old standby. I would argue that demanding a demonstration of "substantially equivalent" is not good enough. If it's substantially equivalent, why take a risk? Class III devices should stand up to the same rigorous testing that I am advocating for pharmaceuticals: the demonstration of meaningful efficacy.

The definition of a "device" is rather loose. Not all devices are inorganic gizmos like the hardware used to fuse spines. For example, hyaluran solution was licensed as a device for use in facilitating the insertion of the artificial lens following cataract extraction, but it was licensed as a pharmaceutical to be injected into osteoarthritic knees. Only the latter licensure was based on an RCT; the former was based on observational data and surgical testimony. Hyaluran is a high-molecular-weight sugar molecule that is a constituent of joint fluid, the vitreous humor behind the ocular lens, and the cockscomb. As an aside, hyaluran is far more important as a device used by ophthalmologists when replacing the lens than as a drug used by rheumatologists and orthopedists for joint pain; I don't find the RCTs the slightest bit compelling and never inject these preparations into knees.

There is another aspect of the 1976 amendments that moves devices onto a different regulatory island: the statute essentially preempts any attempt to regulate devices by the states. This bit of legal fine print is not trivial. For example, Charles Riegel lost a suit against Medtronic in a New York court because of this fine print. He underwent a balloon angioplasty in 1996, during which the balloon ruptured, leading to a cardiac arrest, advanced cardiac support, and a coronary artery bypass graft. The patient and his family sued Medtronic, the manufacturer of the angioplasty balloon device. The suit was denied in New York. In our hypothetical case above, Mr. Jones died as a result of the procedure itself but not because of failure of the devices involved.

Poor Mr. Riegel also died; it was his family that appealed the New York court decision. In December 2007 the U.S. Supreme Court heard arguments in *Riegel v. Medtronic*. Jurisdiction was only one of the issues. This suit was revisiting a 1996 Supreme Court decision that FDA licensure and appropriate warnings in labeling did not preclude damages in a medical-device tort. In February 2008 the Supreme Court found 8 to 1 in favor of the manufacturer in *Riegel v. Medtronic*. In effect, device manufacturers have gained tort immunity based on FDA licensure.

In January 2009 a district court in Minnesota expanded the notion that the federal decision preempted state law. The Minnesota suit again involved Medtronic. Is Medtronic liable when the wires (leads) from the Fidelis intracardiac defibrillator break? An intracardiac defibrillator is a device that is implanted in the chest wall with wires extending into the heart. The device monitors the heart rhythm for sudden death and automatically shocks the heart if such occurs. If the wires break, the device is useless, and the patient again is at risk from sudden death from a lethal cardiac rhythm. The Minnesota court found that since the FDA licensed the defibrillator, it was to be assumed that it was licensing its components. Therefore, the FDA approval provides immunity against product-liability suits.

I am not alone in my concern regarding whether FDA approval of devices is an adequate remedy for inadequate devices. So even if our Mr. Jones had died because of failure of the angioplasty balloon and not failure of the angioplasty procedure, Mrs. Jones could not bring a product-liability suit. She also could not bring a malpractice suit against Dr. Clayton, since his diagnosis and treatment was the standard of care in his community. Her lawsuit related to the deceptive nature of the permission slip. Given the gentle nature of the regulation of angioplasty and stents, the fact that no benefit can be demonstrated despite multiple RCTs does not preclude their marketing in the first place.

Angioplasty catheters and stents are not the only devices licensed for no good reason. Take the procedures done through fiberoptic scopes just mentioned as an example of a technological triumph. They are indeed a procedural triumph, but they have downsides. One of the most common of these procedures removes the diseased gall bladder using surgical instruments inserted through small incisions in the abdominal wall and guiding them by direct observation through a laparoscope, a fiberoptic scope also inserted into the abdominal cavity. The procedure, laparoscopic cholecystectomy, is far gentler in every way compared to the classical surgical removal of a diseased gall bladder, the "open" cholecystectomy. The indications for removing the gall bladder are exquisitely well defined and are a classic chapter in the annals of evidence-based medicine. These indications were largely adhered to in the era of the open cholecystectomy, but clearly they are not adhered to any longer. Far more cholecystectomies are performed by laparoscopy than surgeons ever found reason to do before.

The most plausible explanation for this is that the availability of the gentler, more-expedient laparoscopic procedure predisposes surgical judgment toward marginal indications if not unnecessary procedures. This is akin to "off-label" uses of pharmaceuticals. Almost as disconcerting is the loss of the surgical skills to do the old procedure. Laparoscopic cholecystectomies can have complications, including the inadvertent cutting of a blood vessel or bowel. The remedy is to quickly abandon the laparoscopic technique, cut open the abdomen, and repair the damage. Many young laparoscopic surgeons have limited experience doing open surgery in this part of the abdomen. No one should ever think that laparoscopic surgery should be performed without a really good, scientifically based reason.

In the case of laparoscopic cholecystectomy, there are clear-cut indications and unequivocal benefits. Then there's the arthroscope. It's open season on the American knee, and they're gearing up for the shoulder.

Knee Arthroscopy Only Works
if You Want It to Work

Over the course of the next five years, most of us will experience regional knee pain lasting weeks to months. Without anything special happening, we will notice pain in a knee when we bear weight. Walking will be unpleasant, walking quickly very unpleasant, and jogging may be out of the question. We might even limp. Climbing stairs is difficult, but not as difficult as descending them. There is prompt relief sitting or lying down. The knee might seem tight, even swollen, but not warm or so painful we can't bend it at all. Sometimes it feels as if it might give way. Fortunately, if it wasn't for this damnable knee pain, we'd be as well as ever. What to do?

Some will carry on as best they can until their perseverance is rewarded by regression of symptoms. Some seek relief in the over-the-counter remedies about which marketing has made us all keenly aware. Some will turn to purveyors of help—and there are many of these with many kinds of treatments, with and without licensure. Every purveyor will approach your knee pain brandishing the language that derives from their beliefs as to the reason the knee hurts and upon which their treatment is based. When we are hurting, we all become quick studies. Usually, we will get better. When we do, the conclusion that the treatment was effective is inescapable. It matters little that nearly all the particulars of these treatments, the "modalities," have been studied systematically and found to have no specific beneficial effect. We will return time and again when faced with the next episode of regional knee pain, or backache, or whatever to purchase another dose of the language of treatment and the adjunctive physical, manual, dietary, pharmaceutical, or spiritual modality. We will revisit this phenomenon in detail in chapter 6.

In our culture, the top of this therapeutic pyramid is occupied by the most technically based, usually invasive, potentially dangerous, and expensive treatments. Some patients head straight for the top; others limp up only when their knee pain persists despite alternatives. Near the top are the doctors who are willing to inject something into your painful knee. They brandish the most marginal scientific support of effectiveness, whether its hyaluran or cortisone or whatever. At the summit, decorated and highly rewarded, are the surgeons who are trained to fix the knee.

Each year, over 5 million people seek the care of American orthopedic surgeons for knee pain. All these patients are subjected to an examination of the knee that involves various yankings and pullings handed down from generation to generation of orthopedists despite the modern science that renders nearly all the "findings" nonspecific—meaning they correlate very poorly with knee anatomy. Nearly all of these patients undergo an X-ray examination despite the fact that nearly all findings, including osteoarthritis and spurs, are also nonspecific—meaning they are common findings in knees that are not hurting and likely to be present in your knee before it started to hurt and after it stops. Nearly all undergo magnetic resonance imaging (MRI), which may demonstrate damage to ligaments and other structures in the knee ("ACL" tears, torn menisci, etc.). You get the idea: these, too, are nonspecific and highly likely to be present in your other knee or in the hurting knee when it stops hurting or the knees of many who are walking and jogging today. But Americans expect to be diagnosed. More and more, orthopedists are aggregating in partnerships in the specialty hospitals they own in which all the profitable diagnostic and therapeutic paraphernalia are convenient. The American health-care system considers this evolution an example of efficiency that promotes quality and saves money. The surgeons love it.

Science or no science, it is difficult for a surgeon, and more difficult for a patient, to see a damaged structure in the knee without ascribing the knee pain to that structure and fearing for the future. Furthermore, if the damage is reparable, shouldn't it be fixed? Such reasoning induced a generation of orthopedic surgeons to offer their services in removing torn menisci by cutting open the knee. It took quite a while for patients to recover from the procedure, but most did. Most also have damaged knees when followed up decades later. Was the damage a result of whatever led to the tearing of the menisci in the first place or to the surgery? We don't know. We do know that removing torn menisci by opening the knee is no solution in the long run.

Along came arthroscopic surgery. Torn menisci can be removed, damaged cartilage smoothed out, and other ligaments repaired through tubes inserted into the knee using three small incisions. Recovery is rapid. The technology is no more impressive than that involved in laparoscopic procedures; the hand-eye coordination required is impressive, though less so than many a modern video game. Over 500,000 knees are subjected to invasion by arthroscopes each year. It is the commonest elective orthopedic procedure in America. Most patients are grateful and bear the stigmata—the three little scars—as a sign of triumph. Arthroscopy is certainly responsible for a great transfer of wealth, but any certainty as to specific benefit has been called into question by randomized controlled trials.

One RCT was from the Veterans Administration Hospital in Houston and published in 2002. Patients with pain in a knee ascribed to cartilage damaged by osteoarthritis received the three small incisions. In only half, the arthroscope was inserted into the knee and the osteoarthritis surgically treated. The patients were not aware of whether they underwent arthroscopic surgery or the sham procedure. There was no significant difference in outcome. Another trial, performed in Canada, was published in 2008. It was similar, except instead of a sham procedure, the patients received "conservative" care, including physical modalities. Over the course of two years, the surgery did not offer any advantage. There are also observational studies, mainly from Europe, comparing arthroscopic surgery with conservative care for a number of putative knee tragedies, including the ACL and other ligament tears, where the procedure is more extensive and recovery prolonged. You're as likely to get better in terms of function and comfort if you forego the surgery. And I suspect, when this all plays out, your knee will be better off in the long run without the three surgical stigmata.

A Canadian- or European-style trial would not come up with the same result in the United States. Most patients in the United States are burdened with the preconception that the surgery must be better because it fixed the osteoarthritis. In the United States, one needs a sham surgical control group to overcome the bias of preconception. Once an American hears there's something structurally wrong that can be fixed, few are able to mobilize the patience to let the knee heal on its own, even though we know arthroscopic surgery cannot be shown to offer the patient's knee any specific advantage. The American orthopedic community is quick to explain that they reserve their arthroscopic surgery for patients with different causes of knee pain and that they are particularly adept at choosing the patients with osteoarthritis likely to be helped. They learned this response from interventional cardiologists who are similarly wedded to their stents.

My response to these arthroscopists is the same I offered the interventional cardiologists: *show me* with well-executed, randomized, sham-controlled trials that you can identify the subset that is advantaged by your devices and that others can utilize your criteria to identify them as well. Until then, I will inform my patient as to the state of the science. I will assure him that it is reasonable if he simply does the best he can to get on with it, try an exercise bicycle or water aerobics, and be patient. This too shall pass. And I will ask the Citizen Patient to reflect on whether the fashion in which the FDA regulates devices begs revision.

When Is a Picture NOT Worth a Thousand Words?

There is no bright side to the nuclear disasters at Fukushima, Chernobyl, Three-Mile Island, Nagasaki, Hiroshima, or any slightly lesser instances of nuclear ignominy. When will we ever learn? It's not just the citizen that needs to understand ionizing radiation; it's also the Citizen Patient.

We live our lives engulfed in waves of electromagnetic particles. These waves have an enormous range of frequencies and, at each frequency, an enormous range of intensity. The energy of the wave is determined by its frequency. Low-frequency waves are composed of particles (quanta or photons) that are relatively low in energy. While the lower-energy electromagnetic waves are ubiquitous, we are unaware of most of them; radio waves and the static fields around power lines are examples of electromagnetic waves that do not alter our biology in any discernible or measurable fashion. If these waves are intense enough, however, measurable changes occur, such as the static field from the enormous magnets we use in MRI machines. This field causes the nuclei of some molecules to transiently release heat, which is detected as the MR image. Some other lower-energy waves, such as microwaves, can cause thermal injury if they are intense enough. Visible light is a bit higher in energy, so that it causes a photochemical reaction in the retina at the back of the eye (which is processed as a visual image by our brain). If the light is intense enough, it can cause thermal injury (sunburn). The light from the sun contains higher-energy waves that, fortunately, are filtered by the atmosphere, with the exception of some waves in the near-ultraviolet spectrum.

If the particles in these waves interact with cells in the skin, they have sufficient energy to break up molecules, knocking electrons off the molecule and thereby ionizing it. This creates reactive new molecules—free radicals—that can damage other molecules in the neighborhood, including DNA. Such near-ultraviolet radiation is the least energetic of ionizing radiation. Fortunately, the body has myriad mechanisms to avoid or repair the damage caused by ionizing radiation incurred through sun exposure. There are cells in the skin that make pigment to absorb the electromagnet waves; we call that "tanning" when the skin darkens in response to photo exposure. More important, there are biochemical mechanisms to neutralize free radicals and repair the damage they may have wreaked inside any given cell.

In the case of the skin, this works pretty well for nearly all of us most of our lives. Many folks incur damage to a cell that escapes the repair mechanisms, so that the cell continues to divide longer than normal without losing the need to stay in its home turf. This tends to occur frequently later in life, when the cells heap up as actinic keratoses and basal cell carcinomas. If the cell loses the biological constraints that require home turf, it can spread or metastasize and kill. Hence, a nonpigmented cell can morph into a squamous cell carcinoma. For pigmented cells, the transition is from a freckle to a malignant melanoma. Fortunately, whereas we all are experiencing damage to our skin from ionizing radiation, the protective and repair mechanisms are a match for most of us with most intensities of photo exposure. Nonetheless, rather than simply hope the repair mechanisms are a match, we advise sunscreens designed to block the component of visible light that includes ionizing radiation.

Ionizing radiation from sun exposure is a tiny fraction of the spectrum of ionizing radiation to which we are normally exposed. Slightly more energetic are the particles in medical X-rays. We are exposed to the particles that are emitted from the decay of naturally occurring radioactive substances. We are exposed to the particles in cosmic rays that come from outer space. Clearly, the body's repair mechanisms are a match for nearly all of this for much of our life. As I detail in *Rethinking Aging*, though, all octogenarians are harboring cancer that one can postulate reflects the gradual waning of the repair mechanisms over decades of exposure to ionizing radiation and other carcinogens. There is a theory that suggests a much more dynamic form of homeostasis—radiation hormesis—that postulates that low levels of ionizing radiation are important in stimulating repair mechanisms.

The degree to which these exposures are harmful depends on the intensity of exposure, which is not always a reflection of the intensity emanating from the source. For example, some ionizing radiation can be blocked by paper or aluminum foil, but if the source is incorporated into body chemistry—in a radioactive water molecule (tritiated water), for example—it can do its damage from within the cell. For tritiated water, the effect lasts many years, whereas radioactive iodine molecules captured in the thyroid decay in a week or two. The most dramatic exposures are from high-intensity sources, either by design (radiation therapy for cancer, nuclear weapons) or by accident. High-intensity ionizing radiation destroys rapidly dividing cells first, such as the lining of the gastrointestinal tract (vulnerable from mouth to anus) and the blood-forming cells in bone marrow. If one survives, the lining of the gastrointestinal tract and the bone marrow can regenerate. The lining cells seem little worse for wear, but the bone marrow cells have molecular scars that place them at great risk for leukemia over time.

In the case of accidental exposure, we learned this from the life stories of the survivors of Hiroshima and Nagasaki. We also learned this from the life stories of young people treated for lymphoma, a cancer of the lymph glands. For some forms of lymphoma, Hodgkin's lymphoma in particular, a combination of radiation therapy and chemotherapy can induce long-term remission if not cure. However, decades later, some patients develop leukemia. This is a reasonable trade-off—decades of health for early death—but it is also a reproach to the science. Many of the chemotherapy drugs are "radiomimetic," meaning they are chemicals that behave like ionizing radiation in cells. We need a better way to treat cancer.

The reason I am belaboring radiation biology is to demystify diagnostic radiology. In 1895 Wilhelm Röntgen, Ph.D., was experimenting with running electric current through vacuum tubes when he observed a novel ray, an X-ray. His experiments rapidly led to the visualization of the bones in his wife's hand, the first Nobel Prize in Physics, and a revolution in medical diagnostics. For over fifty years, everyone was enamored with X-rays. Most general practitioners and dentists had their own X-ray machine, which they used at will. Retail shoe stores had adapted fluoroscopes, X-ray boxes to stand on so you could see the bones of your feet in the shoe and gauge fit. By the middle of the twentieth century, everyone thought of X-rays as a form of photography that exposed film to X-rays instead of light. Radiation oncology was in its infancy, and "cobalt" machines were just making their appearance.

Radiobiology was also in its infancy, but that changed rapidly with the development of the atomic bomb. Much that I've discussed above and much more about ionizing radiation has been understood for decades. When I was a clinical associate doing research at the National Institutes of Health in the early 1970s, we were required to take a course in radiobiology that included all the elements necessary to understand the potential for diagnostic imaging to do harm. To this day, much of this is subjugated to diagnostic zeal. Diagnostic radiology flies two banners: Don't you want to know what's there? Don't you want to know what's not there? Doctors of medicine, chiropractic, osteopathy, dentistry, and podiatry all subscribe to this formulation, and their patients have come to expect it. Many years ago, the U.S. Army did the following experiment. Soldiers who attended sick call with regional low back pain were randomized to getting an X-ray of their low back or not. We have long known that such radiographs offer no useful diagnostic information and a lot that is irrelevant. Nothing about the groups differed in follow-up, except the soldiers who were spared the X-ray on base went off base and found someone to X-ray them.

Medical exposure to diagnostic ionizing radiation was a fact of life twenty-five years ago. Few complaints were heard that did not lead to an X-ray, particularly in the context of urgent care. Screening programs, mammography in particular, were promulgated without consideration of the inherent risks—a trade-off that is hardly justifiable, as we will discuss in chapter 5. For some radiographs, the risk from ionizing radiation is trivial. That's particularly true for studies of body parts with little bone marrow or studies where the dose needed for accurate films is low. Examples of the former are X-rays of hands and feet, and examples of the latter are chest X-rays where increasing the dose leads to less definition. Never is the issue much ado about nothing.

The issue escalated twenty-five years ago with the introduction of computerized tomography (CT or CAT) imaging. This is a truly remarkable technological advance allowing for extraordinary definition of body parts. In principle, it is straightforward. Instead of a single source of X-rays going through a body part, multiple sources are focused to image sequential slices of the part. The multiple images are integrated by com-

TABLE 5. The Number of Routine Chest X-Rays or Mammograms That Would Provide as Much Hazard from Ionizing Radiation as a Routine CT Scan

ROUTINE CT SCAN	EQUIVALENT NUMBER OF CHEST X-RAYS	EQUIVALENT NUMBER OF MAMMOGRAMS
Of head	30	5
Of chest	117	20
Of abdomen-pelvis	220	37

Source: Adapted from Rebecca Smith-Bindman and others, "Radiation Dose Associated with Common Computed Tomography Examinations and the Associated Lifetime Attributable Risk of Cancer," *Archives of Internal Medicine* 169, no. 22 (2009): 2078–86.

puter into a highly detailed image of the body part. The resolution can be down to the lumen of blood vessels coursing through the chest, which are barely visible, string-like shadows on the usual chest X-ray. Furthermore, there are modifications that can further enhance the definition of soft tissues throughout the body. The result is a definition of anatomy and pathology as elegant as, if not more elegant than, what one can get from many a routine autopsy. Seldom can one look at a routine X-ray and not wonder if something is missed because of the limited sensitivity.

The result is that CT scans have come to supplant plane radiographs in many clinical settings. In the United States, over 20,000 are performed daily and over 70 million annually in the quest for as much information as possible. Only recently have questions been raised as to the utility of all this information and the risk of the attendant ionizing radiation. An editorial and two surveys were published in the December 2009 issue of the *Archives of Internal Medicine* that are daunting if not horrifying as regards the risks. For example, it is clear that the number of CT orders varies from place to place dramatically, and so does the radiation dose from machine to machine. That speaks to a lack of standardization both in indications for the study and in the way machines are actually used.

The greater difficulty is that a CT image of the chest is equivalent in exposure to ionizing radiation of over a hundred chest X-rays at once. That's a lot of ionizing radiation on radiosensitive tissue in the bone marrow of the ribs and spine. It's even worse for an abdominal CT, as is apparent in Table 5. Radiobiology has gone to great lengths to learn how to convert exposure to ionizing radiation into the risk of cancer. This requires both a consideration of the dose and a consideration of the particular targeted tissue. As mentioned, some tissues are far more sensitive to the malignant effects of ionizing radiation. For example, brain tissue itself is

TABLE 6. Projected Number of Future Cancers That Could Be Related to CT Scans Performed in the United States in 2007

ROUTINE CT SCANS PERFORMED PER YEAR	PREDICTED NUMBER OF RADIATION-INDUCED CANCERS (WOMEN/MEN)	PERCENTAGE OF THE TOTAL NUMBER OF CANCERS ATTRIBUTABLE TO CT EXPOSURE
Head (18.7 million)	1,900/2,100	14
Chest (7.1 million)	3,100/1,000	14
Abdomen-pelvis (18.3 million)	8,500/5,500	48

Source: Adapted from Amy Berrington de Gonzalez and others, "Projected Cancer Risks from Computed Tomographic Scans Performed in the United States in 2007," *Archives of Internal Medicine* 169, no. 22 (2009): 2071–77.

not particularly radiosensitive, but the CT scan exposes much more than the substance of the brain to ionizing radiation, and CTs of the head are exceedingly common for indications as divergent as headache to head trauma with multiple sclerosis and much else thrown in as well. Likewise, CT scans of the abdomen and pelvis are also exceedingly common—again because belly pain seldom escapes the urgent-care setting without one.

Table 6 offers many insights into this complexity. Notice that women are more likely than men to undergo chest and abdominal-pelvic CT studies and receive the greater share of the risk for cancer as a result. It is estimated that 29,000 excess cancers will result from the CT exposure in 2007, and that excludes people who were scanned after a diagnosis of cancer and those performed in the last five years of life. If you assume 50 percent mortality from these radiation-induced cancers, that's about 15,000 people who die before their time. Some of this toxicity can be blunted by making sure that the machines were delivering the minimum amount of ionizing radiation necessary to result in an accurate image. Regulations to accomplish this are forthcoming. Much more can be blunted through attention to evidence regarding the utility of CT scans in particular settings. For example, the science says the yield of important information from a head CT following blunt trauma without loss of consciousness is very low. Or the yield of a CT of the lumbar spine for regional low back pain is worse than low; it leads to misinformation and misinterpretation and increases the risk for unnecessary surgery.

Citizen Patients should not be faced with yet another scenario requiring a query as to "Is this necessary?" or, better yet, "How likely is it that this CT scan can be used to my advantage?" We have the science to define the indications for such tests and to stop underwriting their abuse.

The imaging community is divided into camps that are at each other's throats. The CT radiologists are hangdog given the potential for their machines to do harm, the variability in the use of their machines site to site, and the variability in the dosing site to site. But these are expensive machines that have proliferated across the nation. New, better versions appear all the time. And CT is the turf of a segment of highly paid radiologists, many of whom specialize in particular body parts. They are proclaiming the machines too valuable to have downtime. After all, how can one turn one's back on an exquisite definition of pathology or lack thereof? They have competition from their colleagues who run the even-more-expensive MRI suites. Patients are spared ionizing radiation during an MRI, although if a contrasting dye like gadolinium is injected to enhance definition, serious complications can result. MRI of soft tissue is more exquisite than CT imaging, though CT imaging has the advantage with bones and gives MRI a race for its costliness by injecting various materials that enhance soft-tissue definition. Neither procedure is a pleasure, though many find MRIs intolerably claustrophobic. When push comes to shove, the MRI folks are laying claim to value because of safety. Although ionizing radiation is not an issue, we are assuming on theoretical grounds that there are no long-term hazards of exposure to such an intense magnetic field.

The turf battles will rage until a more important debate supersedes. It is crucial that everyone realizes we have no need to get any image unless we know how to interpret it to the advantage of our patients. MRIs and CT scans share the same precarious perch in this regard. As for the radiologists who are jockeying PET scanners, with rare exception, demonstrable clinical utility is wanting. This is a research tool.

Type II Medical Malpractice

The type of medical malpractice with which we are all familiar I call Type I. That is when a necessary clinical procedure is performed poorly and the outcome is untoward. Type I Medical Malpractice is often contentious when there is doubt as to whether the untoward outcome could have been avoided. After all, modern medicine at its finest is not a match for the course of many a disease process. Furthermore, the clinical arena is complex and often unpredictable, so that errors can occur despite the best of intentions. Studies of the likelihood of a malpractice lawsuit suggest that "best intentions" is an explanation that rests far more easily with patients and their families if the relationship with the physician has some if not all of the qualities I advocate in chapter 8. In times of grief or sadness, all of us are better served by trusting relationships than by the pain that is associated with recrimination. Comforting, caring, and mutual respect are palliative and laudable whenever such are warranted.

Some errors are only apparent; they are not truly errors of commission or omission. These are often reflections of desperation and account for much of the compendium that has captured the media and struck fear in the hearts of Americans about the safety of their hospitals. In our culture, one should not die without putting up a battle. In my last book, *Rethinking Aging*, I explored the downsides of this approach to terminal illness so that we might not fear death to the extreme of making death unnecessarily horrible. But our society expects its physicians to do all they can until there is nothing left to do—and then proclaim defeat with "Do not resuscitate" or another catchphrase. Hence, in the face of desperate illnesses, drugs that might help can be pushed to toxicity, and procedures that might offer little likelihood of benefit in other settings become the symbol of heroics. The outcome is labeled a medical error whenever the doctor caused harm. But as I said, these are not truly errors of commission; these are errors in perspective.

That being said, I am a strident advocate for ready recourse for instances of Type I Medical Malpractice whenever there is malfeasance, and nearly as strident when overt carelessness or hubris are at play. There should be a price to pay, but it should not be paid by the victim, and in the American tort system, the victim is at great risk—at greater risk than the perpetrator. The perpetrator might suffer some stigmatization, but in many circles that is considered the "price of doing business" and fades rapidly into history. But the victim is likely to suffer lifelong scars as a result of bringing a malpractice suit in addition to whatever "scars" precipitated the suit. That's because the American tort system is driven by the degree to which the victim is not made whole again. Many stakeholders stand to lose if the victim regains full health: the attorneys on both sides lose income, the insurance companies cannot justify escalating premiums, and the health-care providers of every ilk involved in clinical recourse, valuing loss, and the determination of residual disability lose their *raison d'être* sooner. The poor victim is under a subliminal if not overt pressure designed to enhance his or her illness perceptions.

The determination that an untoward outcome is the result of an act of Type I Medical Malpractice is often obvious. Sometimes there is a debate as to the likelihood of the untoward outcome regardless of the particular medical action or any medical action. This circumstance often arises when there are untoward consequences of fetal distress: was the response of the obstetrician appropriate in performing a timely Caesarian section or not? Torts (lawsuits relating to personal injuries) for Type I Medical Malpractice are often settled out of court and before trial, but not before a good deal of costly posturing on the part of all parties. If they go to trial, one can be sure that much money is at stake. Trials are expensive for all involved, and a plaintiff's attorneys customarily work on a contingency basis—that is, they are paid a sizable cut of the take and are compensated for their expenses if they win, but they foot the bill up front (sometimes requiring the plaintiff to share in the court costs). The "take" is a penalty on the physician for erring and a much larger payment for the fact that the plaintiff is still not whole again. Furthermore, if the residua include persisting pain and suffering, the penalty can have little to do with income loss and much to do with the projection as to the value of the particular degree of loss of well-being. Jury trials are likely to focus on this latter aspect of the tort rather than the validity of the causal inference. Medical malpractice cases often recruit expert testimony but seldom take on a Daubert mantle as to whether the outcome would have happened or could have happened in other circumstances.

Many larger institutions—hospitals and clinics in particular—no longer purchase malpractice insurance for their physicians. The physicians self-insure, thereby saving the overhead costs of a private insurance company. But administrative overhead in this arena pales compared to the overhead that "health" insurance underwrites. The major costs are in processing the claim and payments beyond medical penalties. Although no one is leaping to introduce a Daubert Standard in the courtroom, institutions are starting to establish panels to decide causation and compensation early in the process, long before a tort is joined. Whenever there's a possibility of Type I Medical Malpractice, identified by staff or patients, the case is presented to an independent panel that is usually made up of peers recruited mainly from the community. Hospitals have several similar panels already, including an ethics panel that opines whenever "pull the plug" is considered and the like and an Institutional Review Board (IRB) that reviews the ethical nature of any research proposal placed before it (these are mandatory for studies involving human beings). So a malpractice panel is charged with the issue of causation, and if they find for the patient using a Daubert-like standard, guilt is admitted quickly and fair compensation offered without contest. Institutions that have adopted this mechanism have seen malpractice costs go down, and more important, instances of malpractice decrease as well. In such a setting, malpractice is not a secretive issue but a reproach to community ethics.

Many years ago, I introduced the notion of Type II Medical Malpractice. I define it as doing the unnecessary to a patient, even if the unnecessary is done well. Stents and CABGs are examples we have just visited. I visit many more in my earlier books. Spine surgery gives interventional cardiology a run for Type II poster child, as I detail in *Stabbed in the Back*. And much that is done to patients with cancer deserves the label and will join spine surgery on the poster at the rate ineffective cancer chemotherapy is licensed and its prescription escalates. I will not reiterate or belabor all this here. But Type II Medical Malpractice is a scourge for which the American legal system offers no recourse. To the contrary, since it defines malpractice as a practice that does not reach the standard of care in the community, most examples of Type II Medical Malpractice cannot qualify as malpractice by the legal standard. Since every interventional cardiologist in the community is immersed in Type II Medical Malpractice, Type II is the standard of care. It's the same flaw in reasoning that has tripped up the movement for enhancing the quality of care in American hospitals. The criteria for quality often are elements of the process of caring for cardiac patients, elements that cannot be shown to be substantially efficacious in RCTs. Hence, improvement in "quality" becomes uniformity in ineffective practices and not improvement in patient well-being.

Common practice as the gold standard is out of date for Type I Medical Malpractice and irrelevant to Type II Medical Malpractice. We need something like the Daubert Standard outside of the courtroom so that we can be better informed by the introduction of the relevant science. Type II Medical Malpractice would be less of an issue if ineffective devices were not licensed and new procedures had to be submitted to RCTs before widespread implementation.

5

Another Good Idea
Still in Waiting

HEALTH PROMOTION, DISEASE PREVENTION

Santé ("to health") and *L'chaim* ("to life") flow readily from our lips. No one is certain of the age or derivation of the term "toast" or the tradition of toasting. There are many explanations, most apocryphal. However, for centuries around the world it has been customary to raise a glass and toast with whomever one is imbibing. Many a toast is in recognition of an event or a person. But the commonest toasts are more generic and fall into four categories:

1. The toast to good luck: *Prost* (German), *Noroc* (Romanian).
2. The general celebratory toast: Cheers (United States), Cheerio (Australia).
3. The toast to the act of drinking: Bottoms up (United States) and the similar sentiment of *Kampai* (Japan), *Skol/Skål* (Sweden and Norway), and *Ganbei* (Mandarin).
4. The toast to health or longevity (by far the commonest): *Salud* (Spanish), *Salute* (Italian), *Santé* (French), *Sláinte* (Gaelic), *be ṣaḥtak* (Arabic), *L'chaim* (Hebrew), *Mabuhay* (Tagalog), *Salam ati* (Persian), *Vivat Na zdrowie* (Polish), *Kedves egeszsegere* (Hungarian), and many more.

Toasting health and longevity by ingesting alcohol is a time-honored tradition. Clinical science should give toasting pause in the twenty-first century. Alcohol is a drug—an ancient drug, but a drug nonetheless. This is not a botanical or herb or any other substance one is likely to encounter in the environment. It is an early contribution of biotechnology. Various sources of sugar must be fermented to create alcohol. Residents of the Zagros Mountains (Persia) figured out how to do this in the Stone Age. Mesopotamians slurped beer through a straw. Alcohol was available in China since Paleolithic times, long utilized in ceremonies and as a source of tax revenues for much of the past millennium. No one has considered alcohol a source of nutrition. Everyone has been aware of the price of excess, most decrying drunkenness, some as sinful. The twentieth century brought to light the lethal potential of acute and chronic exposures, the former a cause of most motor vehicle accidents and the latter of damage to liver, nerves, and more. But it is not the toxicity that causes one to raise a glass. In moderation, nearly every culture has enjoyed and valued the taste and the sensation associated with imbibing. It is in this context that a potentially toxic drug is used to toast health and long life.

Would you believe that toasting in this fashion is actually good for your health and longevity? Is it possible that all the toasts to health and to life for all these millennia increased the likelihood of health and longer life? Is it possible that all the toasts to good luck and camaraderie also increased the likelihood of longer life because the ingestion of moderate amounts of alcohol with or without the toasting is salutary in this fashion? There is a scientific literature that suggests as much. There are several long-term community-based studies of health hazards, usually named after their principal setting—Framingham, Massachusetts; Tecumseh, Michigan; Rotterdam, Holland; and others. Most are looking at all sorts of cardiovascular risks, famously at cholesterol. Most have made an interesting observation relating to the consumption of alcohol: people who drink a couple of drinks a day live longer than those who drink more—or less. I'll drink to that. In order to infer such a relationship from the large cohorts of community residents they follow for decades, the scientists go to great lengths to be certain that nothing else they know of accounts for this relationship. For example, maybe either avoiding alcohol or more liberal consumption of it causes diabetes or hypertension or some other confounder that thwarts longevity. These possibilities are explored and compensated for in the design of the statistical analysis of the data. They still come up with no better explanation than a couple of drinks are better for you than more or less. This is the classic U-shaped relationship seen with many of the cardiovascular risk factors associated with health-adverse behaviors: body mass index, blood pressure, glucose metabolism, cholesterol, and others. The observation has led to a wealth of theories about the biochemistry that sharpens both edges of alcohol's sword.

Skeptical? I've led you down this garden path so that I could point out the brambles. Could it be that all these epidemiologists and biostatisticians were missing something that correlated with alcohol consumption but better explained the U-shaped curve? Of course it could. Every epidemiologist worth her salt fears the confounder(s) that were not measured or could not be measured. The literature of causation is littered with associations that were trashed when a stronger association was discerned.

Who drinks a couple of drinks a day, a cocktail or two, but not more and not less? Could this be a marker of a more-advantaged lifestyle? Could alcohol consumption be a surrogate measure of one's station in society? Is this the confounder that so many epidemiologists neglected to take into consideration all these years? Could something about one's status in one's ecosystem be more determinative of when one dies—of all-cause mortality—than any element of daily living?

The answer is a compelling, unavoidable, resounding *yes*. Believing this answer is difficult in a society that has been nurtured on the negative answer. Applying this answer to one's worldview runs headlong into society's investment in the reductionistic alternative. We are taught that we are the sum of our parts, and that attention to each in turn is the secret to health and longevity. We must eat "well," exercise "well," stay thin, and ingest all sorts of pharmaceuticals to keep the grim reaper at bay. We have been misled. This is the most important lesson the Citizen Patient must learn if the approach to his health and the health of the public in the twenty-first century is to be enlightened.

"Toasting health" is an object lesson. Table 7 presents the results of one of the studies demonstrating the U-shaped curve of the association between alcohol consumption and mortality. The data upon which this is based is the Health and Retirement Study, a long-term study of a representative sample of U.S. adults who were at least fifty-five years old when the study population was recruited. The first row of data is the observed mortality over the course of four years. It is remarkable that 14 percent of those who never drank alcohol died, as did a similar percentage (12 percent) of those who imbibed the equivalent of three drinks per day. But half as many whose consumption was intermediate died. That means that the odds of dying are reduced by 50 percent—that is, the odds of dying (odds ratio) if you ingest a drink a day compared to abstinence is 0.5. This

TABLE 7. Confounders of the Association between Alcohol Consumption and Four-Year Mortality

ADJUSTING OBSERVED MORTALITY OF CONFOUNDERS	NONDRINKER (NUMBER OF SUBJECTS [N] = 5,672)	<1 DRINK PER WEEK (N = 2,327)	<1 DRINK PER DAY (N = 1,901)	1 DRINK PER DAY (N = 1,691)	2 DRINKS PER DAY (N = 550)	3 DRINKS PER DAY (N = 378)
Observed mortality (percentage)	14	10	7	7	8	12
Adjusted for demographics (age, sex, race)	Reference	0.80 (.067–0.94)	0.56 (0.46–0.69)	0.50 (0.40–0.62)	0.65 (0.47–0.90)	0.96 (0.68–1.35)
Adjusted for demographics plus risk factors (comorbidities, smoking, obesity)	Reference	0.93 (0.78–1.10)	0.67 (0.54–0.83)	0.57 (0.46–0.72)	0.67 (0.47–0.94)	1.03 (0.72–1.47)
Adjusted for demographics plus psychosocial factors (support, depression, religion)	Reference	0.91 (0.77–1.08)	0.68 (0.55–0.83)	0.60 (0.48–0.75)	0.75 (0.53–1.05)	1.01 (0.71–1.44)
Adjusted for demographics plus socioeconomic status	Reference	0.91 (0.77–1.08)	0.69 (0.56–0.84)	0.62 (0.50–0.77)	0.77 (0.55–1.07)	1.09 (0.77–1.53)
Adjusted for all of the above plus functional limitations	Reference	1.06 (0.89–1.28)	0.85 (0.68–1.06)	0.72 (0.57–0.91)	0.79 (0.55–1.11)	1.11 (0.77–1.60)

Source: Adapted from S. J. Lee, R. L. Sudore, B. A. Williams, and others, "Functional Limitations, Socioeconomic Status, and All-Cause Mortality in Moderate Alcohol Drinkers," *Journal of the American Geriatrics Society* 57 (2009): 955–62.

is the raw data in the first row. The rows that follow are the results of statistical models that take into account potential confounders, or the other factors that might explain this relationship better than alcohol consumption. The results of such an analysis are expressed as an "odds ratio." The numbers in parentheses are the 95 percent confidence interval, the range that one can be 95 percent confident captures the odds ratio. So if the odds ratio is 0.7 and the 95 percent confidence interval is 0.5 to 0.9, you can be quite confident that the risk is reduced somewhere between 50 percent and 10 percent. If the range crosses 1.0, one is bucking the odds to assume that the odds ratio is different from the abstinence reference. If the range crosses 1.0, the safe assumption is that it makes no difference.

The next row takes into account the demographics of the population: age, sex, and ethnicity. This does not alter the observed U-shaped relationship between alcohol consumption and mortality. The third row takes into account the influence of demographics along with conventional risk factors, such as the presence of other important diseases (comorbidities) as well as health-adverse behaviors. Apparently, these additional confounders make a difference; if they were not present, the difference between the reference anchor and the moderate drinkers would be reduced by 10 percent. This is also the magnitude of influence of psychosocial confounders and, separately, lower socioeconomic status. If one takes the influence of the combination of comorbidities, psychosocial confounders, and reduced socioeconomic status (the bottom row), the U-shaped relationship between alcohol consumption and mortality essentially becomes flat. There is no influence of this range of exposure to alcohol on all-cause mortality. We were fooled by not realizing the importance of the socioeconomic and psychosocial confounders.

Proximate-Cause Epidemiology

We are often fooled, and the "we" is not simply a gullible public. The mainstream of modern epidemiology and biostatistics continues to miss this forest for the trees. Epidemiology emerged from relative obscurity in the 1960s with biostatistics as its handmaiden in response to legislation mandating the demonstration of efficacy for licensing drugs. Prior to that, epidemiology was largely the purview of the public-health establishment and traditionally harnessed to sort out the cause of epidemics (hence "epidemiology"). As for biostatistics, probability theory was the purview of mathematicians. Some epistemologists who were concerned with the differences between inductive and deductive reasoning dabbled in statistics. Inductive reasoning takes the world as we see it and attempts to make sense of it. Deductive reasoning is the testing of any hypothesis derived from inductive reasoning, as in a randomized controlled trial (RCT) of a pharmaceutical. In the past half century, however, epidemiology, biostatistics, and considerations of inductive versus deductive reasoning have emerged from obscurity. They are a major emphasis of schools of public health and of the entire "translational research" establishment, which seeks to demonstrate a role in patient care for any scientific insight.

Faced with the mandate to probe the efficacy of pharmaceuticals, the way forward for epidemiology and biostatistics required reductionism. The most efficient and sensitive approach demanded a study design that recruited similar people and tested outcomes that could be quantified in a relatively short period of time. As a result, we have accumulated a wealth of information about the biology of particular, discrete bodily functions and structures in health and disease. We have come to know a lot about the kidney, the heart, the knee, particular blood vessels, the liver, particular blood cells, and so much more in the fifty years since I entered medical school. Certainly, many of these structures are critical; but more important, this reductionistic approach fosters the assumption that we are but the sum of all these parts, and understanding them individually offers great insights into the human predicament. Hence, we have a great deal of information about disease-specific outcomes, such as the likelihood of dying from heart disease or stroke or renal failure. This is called "proximate-cause epidemiology." It is the study of the diagnosis on our death certificates. Thanks to proximate-cause epidemiology, we also know a lot about the hazards that predispose us to a particular illness or to death from a particular disease. That's how we came to know all the U-shaped curves for risk factors like blood sugar and cholesterol, blood pressure, heftiness, and the like.

This is the basis for public-health "prevention" agendas that urge, even coerce, us to reduce these risk factors at all cost with the expectation that doing so will promote our well-being. This is also the rationale for the enormous effort by the pharmaceutical industry to "discover" and purvey generation after generation of drugs, each more costly than the last, to reduce our risk factors. Likewise, this is the rationale for complementary industries purveying all sorts of dietary combinations and concoctions purported to have similarly salutary effectiveness. In *Worried Sick* and *Rethinking Aging*, I examine the science that demonstrates how ineffective nearly all this activity has proved. We have been more than misled by proximate-cause epidemiology; we have been brainwashed. Furthermore, we have accepted an enormous transfer of wealth in a misguided approach to preventing disease and promoting health.

Life-Course Epidemiology

There is another playing field for modern epidemiology and biostatistics that is far-less-visible and far-less-influential than proximate-cause epidemiology. Many of the players are similarly brilliant, and their contributions in the past fifty years represent similarly important advances. However, these epidemiologists and biostatisticians don't just play on a different playing field; they play in an entirely different league. Generally, each of the two leagues is unwilling to cite the other's literature, let alone cross-fertilize. In Britain, where much of the pioneering work in modern epidemiology was nurtured, this separate league is termed "life-course epidemiology"; in the United States, it's "social epidemiology." I've written extensively about life-course epidemiology in my earlier books, and I've contributed to its literature from the perspective of workplace health. Some of the leading lights include Sir Michael Marmot and Richard Wilkinson in the United Kingdom and Lisa Berkman and George Kaplan in the United States. Life-course epidemiologists do not focus on the immediate cause of death. Rather, life-course epidemiology takes as its premise the inevitability of death and focuses on when it happens, not how. In other words, if I live to a ripe old age, I don't care how many diseases I have or which one is my reaper. I only care that I made it to a ripe old age, that the journey was satisfying and the dying comfortable. Life-course epidemiology studies the journey and its influence on the likelihood of avoiding death from any cause before one's time.

Remember all those U-shaped life-hazard curves like the one illustrated in Table 7, the U-shaped curves for cholesterol, blood sugar, blood pressure, and heft? All of those were formulated by observing populations over time with the preconception that cholesterol, blood sugar, blood pressure, and body mass index were important risk factors for cardiovascular disease and death from cardiovascular disease. All of them are interrelated to such a degree that their coincidence has been labeled the "metabolic syndrome." Today, all of these relationships have been reformulated taking into account measures of socioeconomic status and psychosocial challenges. They remain important mortal hazards at the extremes of the range of values one finds in the general population. But between the extremes, very little hazard remains—too little to warrant a federal case. All of these elements of the metabolic syndrome correlate with various measures of socioeconomic and psychosocial challenge.

For example, if you're poor, you're more likely to die young; and if you're poor, you're more likely to have the metabolic syndrome. But if you're poor and don't have the metabolic syndrome, you're still about as likely to die young as if you're poor and have the metabolic syndrome. The converse holds, as well: if you're not poor, the metabolic syndrome bodes far less evil.

Psychosocial and Socioeconomic Challenges to Reaching a Ripe Old Age

We're not talking about trivial influences. Let's take the easiest measure of socioeconomic status: income. If you're in the lowest quintile (lowest 20 percent), you are likely to die of some disease or other (all-cause mortality) about seven years sooner than folks born the same year as you (your birth cohort) who are in the upper quintiles. Contrast this with cholesterol levels. If you are at or near the highest percent of cholesterol levels, you are likely to die two to three years sooner than the rest of your birth cohort; but if you're not at this extreme—say, you're just in the upper quintile—you have only months of longevity at risk. Some of the malevolence of a life of relative deprivation relates to the attributes of such a lifestyle, such as the proclivity to abuse tobacco and alcohol. But there are many other social factors that don't distribute evenly across the socioeconomic spectrum, factors that include social support and education. A recent systematic review of this literature in the *American Journal of Public Health* (doi: 10.2105/AJPH.2010.300086) by Sandro Galea and colleagues concludes that social factors are at least as important an explanation for all-cause mortality in the United States as any measure of biochemical or behavioral abnormality. When I and others look at this data, we conclude that only some 20 percent of our mortal hazard is captured by traditional disease-focused processes and measures. That is not to trivialize these traditional hazards. I do not trivialize them in my earlier books, although I place our standard remedies under a harsh glare. In this chapter, I discuss the 80 percent that influences longevity, or the age at which one will die from something (all-cause-mortality).

One of the themes of *Rethinking Aging* is the definition of a "ripe old age." If one graphs the change in longevity of the people residing in various resource-advantaged countries through the twentieth century, the result is startling (Figure 5). People are more and more likely to be octoge-

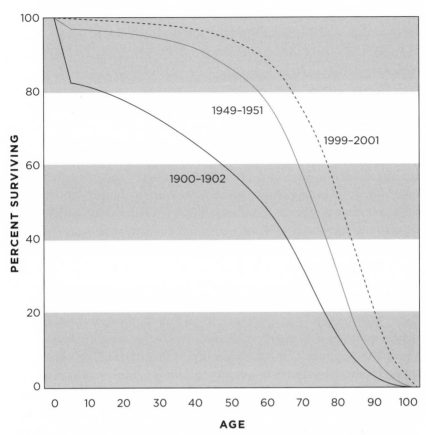

Figure 5. Changes in U.S. longevity rates during the twentieth century. Note how the survival curves become increasingly rectangular as the century progresss. We are ever more likely to become octogenarians, at which point the curves turn increasingly vertical. (Source: U.S. Public Health Service, *National Vital Statistic Reports*, vol. 57, no. 1, August 5, 2008)

narians, but not much more likely to be nonagenarians. It's as if the optimal longevity for our species is close to eighty-five. Ideally, we'd all live to age eighty-five (with some slight variation) and die of something on our eighty-fifth birthday looking back on a pleasing journey. It is important for all of us to realize that the chance of arriving and the quality of the journey are exquisitely linked with our microecology, the world in which we live day by day, and not so dependent on individual elements of that world that we confront day by day. Microecology is a more global notion that can be captured by three interrelated aspects of life. None lends itself to facile definition, but all three need to be recognized and understood by every Citizen Patient so as to avoid misconceptions perpetrated by proximal-cause epidemiology and to take to heart inferences regarding the importance of the structure of the society in which one lives.

For the traditional economist and those involved in health policy, poverty is a measure of purchasing power. The "Poverty Level" is generally defined as three times the amount of money necessary for subsistence. That's a different quantity, depending on the cost of subsistence in a particular locale. But for sociologists, anthropologists, psychologists, and many others, including physicians, poverty is more than an issue in limited purchasing power. It's a station in life, a tenuous station with limited opportunity. It is also associated with limited life expectancy.

But even this relationship is not so straightforward. The degree to which poverty limits longevity depends less on the limits on purchasing power than on the degree to which others in the microecology are not limited in purchasing power. The easiest metric for this relationship is the "income gap," the difference in income between the lowest and highest quintiles in a given population. The bigger the income gap, the sooner the poor die. You can demonstrate this relationship across the resource-advantaged world—country to country, state to state, even district to district in a single urban area like Los Angeles. It has been termed the "Robin Hood Effect" in recognition of the beneficence of a more-uniform income distribution. Hence, the lower-income quintile in the northern Midwest matches the longevity of the lower quintile across the Canadian provinces and exceeds the longevity of the lower quintile in the U.S. South. However, though the lower quintiles in the U.S. South have more purchasing power than the lower quintiles in a country like Greece, the poor in Greece live longer. It has nothing to do with the olive oil. It has something to do with notions of social cohesiveness, with feelings of disaffection.

The biology of the stigma of poverty is tantalizing. Realize that most of the countries in the resource-advantaged world do not support means-based disparities in health care. To the contrary, they offer universal access to health care, and still the Robin Hood effect is manifest. So it's not a matter of health care. The answer lies deeper in human biology. Some of it is in utero; there are long-term studies in Britain that suggest that blunted longevity is imprinted on a fetus born into the lower quintile. But it is not immutable. If you are born into a lower quintile and manage to move up the socioeconomic scale into a higher quintile, your longevity improves, but you never quite catch up with those born into that higher quintile. It can go the other way, too: longevity in Russia dropped by a decade within a decade of the fall of the Berlin Wall with no discernible change in the degree to which the population pursued health-adverse behaviors (such as smoking, excessive alcohol intake, dietary indiscretion, etc.).

We have no good science but lots of appealing theories as to how relative poverty manages to move all-cause mortality toward younger years. It also renders a poor person's years of life less pleasing. This is the population that is more likely to perceive themselves as basically unwell and more likely to find life's many predicaments memorable if not insurmountable. Some of the theories for this pall look to nutrients, even micronutrients. Others are planted in the soft science of "psycho-immunology," which postulates a malignant role for the stressfulness of poverty. There is no reason to think there is a single mechanism. But there is every reason to be aware that the more a population stratifies, the more the poor pay a personal price for the good fortunes of the rich.

JOB SATISFACTION

Of course, the unemployed, underemployed, and poorly paid join the ranks of those facing poverty or relative poverty on the march toward an earlier grave. But life in the workplace has a far-less-obvious grip on our health and longevity.

Do you like your job? Do you feel valued at work? Is your job secure? Understanding the health consequences of a negative response to any of these queries did not come easily. The clue was in the incidence of workers' compensation insurance claims for disabling low back pain. In order to garner a workers' compensation award for a backache, the low back pain must occur in the course of working and be considered a personal injury that arose as a consequence of the demands of tasks that are customary and customarily comfortable. This social construction is one focus of *Stabbed in the Back*.

The "compensable back injury" was invented in the 1930s and has come to dominate thinking about health and safety even in the modern workplace. Furthermore, the notion that a backache, as opposed to a headache, is an "injury" is now the common sense, even though it flies in the face of common experience. Everyone gets backaches—often and repeatedly through life. Most cope so well that the episodes are not even memorable, despite the fact that they always present challenges to function. Some seek medical care, and some seek recourse for a compensable injury.

It makes sense that those who seek recourse do so because the pain is more intense. However, that explains very little. The overwhelming reason people seek recourse is that their menu for coping is truncated, if not depleted, by confounding influences in life at home or at work. When life is not going well, the back pain intensifies. In our culture, we are wont to assume that life is not going well because of the back pain rather than vice versa.

We now have a robust and compelling science to disabuse us of the first assumption and to establish the vice versa as far more likely. In the workplace, the confounders to coping are the drivers to workers' compensation claims for low back "injuries" in all resource-advantaged countries except Japan. When I studied the Japanese system, there was considerable social pressure not to launch a workers' compensation claim for a backache because to do so results in inspections and embarrassment. However, unlike all other countries, the recourse of "sick leave" in Japan is almost as advantaged as recourse under workers' compensation awards and provides an alternative safety valve. Workers' compensation claims for low back pain are the canary in the workplace indicative of individual or group job dissatisfaction.

Much work has been applied to dissecting the notion of "job dissatisfaction." The physical demands of work in the modern workplace, the degree of monotony, and work "architecture" (breaks, shifts, etc.) are not prime movers in rendering a job unsatisfying. Defects in social cohesiveness and social capital predominate. The price one pays for having no option other than a job that must be tolerated goes beyond the disquiet, loathing, stress, unhappiness, and whatever one feels when mired in such an unpleasant circumstance. It goes beyond any tendency to seek comfort in health-adverse behaviors, such as excessive eating or tobacco and alcohol abuse. It is another independent cause of death before one's time from something—all-cause mortality.

The corollary inference has also been tested repeatedly and with increasing frequency. A nurturing job, one that leaves you comfortable in your skin, is salutary. But if someone or some event rattles your cage, it can have dire consequences. The "best" experiments are longitudinal studies of workforces faced with impending outsourcing and workforces following downsizing. These are dialectics that serve to preserve the capital of those with the power to outsource and downsize. They are dialectics championed by Friedrich Hayek (1899–1992), an Austrian economist who immigrated to the United States after World War II. Hayek argued that Keynesian policies to combat unemployment were counterproductive because they caused inflation. Hayek gained a Nobel Prize, and employers gained a powerful weapon. But there's a downside to downsizing. The price is paid in human capital, in the health and longevity of those who are cast aside and, to a measurable though lesser extent, of those who remain. In some of these so-called natural experiments, the financial advantage realized by the employer is counterbalanced by the costs incurred by other agencies that provide whatever the entitlement of the unemployed and the sick. *Stabbed in the Back* offers a detailed discussion of this epidemiology. For our purposes here, realize that the goal of enlightened capitalism is to provide nurturing employment. The price paid otherwise is a society that is stratified between the well and anxious versus the sick and angry.

COMMUNITY

Sociologists have long studied and understood notions of social cohesiveness and social capital. Three intellectual giants said it all *fin de siècle*: David Émile Durkheim (1858–1917) developed notions of social solidarity and the "collective conscience." Max Weber (1864–1917) studied the interplay between secularization and capitalism in the development of twentieth-century Western society. Throw in the work of Karl Marx (1818–83) on the role of the proletariat and you have the essence of the definition of "community" and of "society." The generations of scholars to follow have bandied about, probed, debated, elaborated, and tweaked this definition for the past century. We are a communal species, and the whole of our community is greater than its parts. Furthermore, the complexion of the whole is a reflection of the interactions between the members of the community.

Some of the most compelling science is in the literature on workplace health and safety. A subset of that literature considers "job satisfaction" from the perspective of the workforce and not the individual worker. There is complementary literature looking at the health and safety of community-dwelling elderly people. These literatures are discussed in detail in *Rethinking Aging*. But the inferences generalize broadly, even to colonies of primates. Social isolation and ostracism are lethal. We don't know how this malevolence is meted out, but without a sense of community, one's longevity is compromised. Ayn Rand's Atlas may shrug me off, but he could do so longer if he subjugated self-interest to the greater good, at least to some extent.

I raise my glass "To fulfillment" as the secret to health. Most insist on looking for the secret in health care or risk reduction or both. The risk reducers, whose mantra is "health lifestyle," are joined at the hip with those whose mantra is "green." Their view of the forest is obscured by their preconceptions.

Public Health Policy at the Edge of
Reductio ad Absurdum

ENVIRONMENTAL HAZARDS

Some time ago, I was invited to address the membership of the American Petroleum Institute at its annual meeting in Charleston. My topic related to arm pain in the workplace. The next session was by a panel of scientists and policy wonks confronting proposals by the Environmental Protection Agency to increase the stringency of the regulations regarding ambient benzene concentrations. Benzene is a very simple, basic hydrocarbon, a ring of six carbon atoms (C) each with a hydrogen atom (H) attached:

Benzene is a colorless, volatile, highly flammable constituent of crude oil and the basic building block of all petrochemicals. It is detectable naturally in the environment in our water and atmosphere. It also has been known for nearly a century to be a cause of leukemia. As was the case with ionizing radiation exposure, benzene cannot be wholly eliminated or avoided; it is part of life on this planet, as is an endemic frequency of leukemia. Furthermore, the more we attempt to reduce exposure, the more we compromise the efficiency with which we can utilize petrochemicals. If we eliminated products that require petrochemical-based components, we'd nearly be hunter-gatherers again. Hence, the tension between the public-health community and the petrochemical industry is predictable.

It is anything but dispassionate, however; discussions of benzene exposure rapidly degenerate into a battle of agendas, many of which are hidden and seldom driven solely by considerations of the health of the general public or those particularly prone to exposure. That is not to say there have been no regulatory advances. To the contrary, benzene has been banned as an additive to gasoline, even though it improves octane and the performance of the combustion engine. Workers, including scientists, involved in using petrochemicals must have appropriate protection from exposure. However, to reduce the degree to which the petrochemical industry contaminates the environment to baseline is an enormous and enormously expensive undertaking that would dramatically affect the cost of doing business in many, nearly all, sectors. Hence, the battle over benzene pollution is waged with the statistics of health risk assessment.

Fortunately, this battle is fought over very small effects—very small theoretical changes in the likelihood of leukemia, changes that cannot be measured directly with any likelihood of reproducibility. It's the same issue we considered with drug trials seeking small effects but worse, since one can't ethically do an RCT and experimentally probe for the difference in outcome after high versus low exposures to ambient benzene. One has to settle for observational data and estimates of the degree of exposure over time. Instead of stating this up front, opposing "limits of exposure" are hawked as if they were articles of fact rather than faith. There is no easy way out of this conundrum except to educate the public to ask when this is much ado about nothing meaningful for the health of the public. This is the flip side of our discussion of drug trials. Regardless of the theoretical possibilities, the analysis of observational data should be designed to detect clinically meaningful effects so as to avoid being fooled by trivial, irreproducible noise.

Two forces stand between this degree of maturity and the current tendency toward a scare of the week. One is the kind of honest zeal that borders on zealotry. Far more concerning are the agendas that profit their advocates—those for whom zeal is but a ploy. The public pays the price for both forces in unintended consequences. When creosote products were banned from paint because a carcinogenic potential can be demonstrated following intensive exposures in animal experiments, the only certain effects are that outdoor structures require repainting far more frequently and wealth is transferred from one set of purveyors to the coffers of another.

The current flurry of environmental concern relates to the changing demographics. We've discussed the shift in longevity; various groups are lined up to take credit. I'm aligned with those who look at the structure of society for answers rather than the prowess of the produce or pharmaceutical industries. There is a parallel shift in the age that menopause occurs. No one seems exercised about either of these shifts. Adult height has also been increasing. The social construction holds this to be a good thing, and various components of the nutrition industry vie for honors. But there is also a shift in the age of puberty, particularly female puberty. Menarche (first menstrual period) has been occurring younger and younger with each generation for some time, and this shift may be accelerating, so that "normal" is moving toward age ten.

The shifting age of puberty caught society by surprise. No one was certain whether it was a good or bad thing—until recently. Somehow the notion took hold that we are poisoned by hormones in our environment. Farmers are giving cows hormones, estrogens in particular, that get into our milk. Isn't that bad for us, particularly since we now "know" that hormone-replacement therapy is a problem for adults?* Hence, the "organic" food industry came into being and has flourished. Then scientists demonstrated that there are many chemicals that have estrogen-like effects when tested in the laboratory in test-tube systems. These "xenoestrogens" include BPA, PBBs, and phthalates used in manufacturing plastics; the herbicide atrazine; and toxic chemicals like dioxin and PCBs. Exposures to all of these are regulated in the industrial setting. Accidents happen and corporate scofflaws exist, leading to toxic contamination of the environment that should engender forceful regulatory and punitive responses. But that's not what all the fuss is about. Traces of many of these toxins can be detected in the environment, including in water sources and sometimes foodstuffs. After it was shown that traces of BPA can leach out into the fluids contained in plastic baby bottles, there was near hysteria. Parents rushed to replace these Trojan Horses with glass bottles. We're living longer, aging later, and growing taller. Shouldn't there be galloping cognitive dissonance about the extent of our environmental minefield? If it's a minefield out there, why are we living longer, aging later, and growing taller?

---

*I discuss this at length in *Worried Sick*. It is an object lesson in small effects: trivial risk versus trivial benefit.

While a great segment of the public-health community is committed to finding the mines in the environmental minefield of life, another segment is committed to identifying the hazards that lurk in our bodies. Some of these are stealth diseases that are smoldering below a level that causes symptoms; others are predispositions waiting to be triggered. I touch on the topic of screening in earlier chapters and emphasize it in my previous books. Screening has "face validity"; it makes so much sense that criticism seems inappropriate. However, screening is an exceedingly demanding clinical exercise from a scientific perspective. In order for any screening test to be valuable, it must be accurate; it must seek to detect something that is important to the individual being screened; and if that something is detected, there must be a therapeutic option that leads to a meaningful benefit. In other words, you don't want a screening test unless (1) the result is reliable; (2) the disease or potential disease is important; and (3) we can do something about it.

For the average person—that is, one without a family history of early-life colorectal cancer—one screening flexible sigmoidoscopy at around age sixty is defensible on these grounds. Colorectal cancer grows relatively slowly and predictably. If a cancer is detected, it is likely to be at an early stage and curable by surgery. A colorectal cancer that develops after this screening test is unlikely to cause death before some other disease does that deed. The same considerations resulted in revision of the recommendations for "Pap" smears for cervical cancer. However, most of the screening tests advised by one or several august bodies of experts fail on one or more of the criteria for effectiveness. That includes screening mammography, screening for type 2 diabetes (with many tests, including the HbA1C foisted on the citizens of New York City), screening for "high cholesterol," PSA or digital rectal exams to screen for prostate cancer, and bone mineral density for risk for fragility fractures, to mention a few of the object lessons. None of these screening programs accomplish what everyone assumes they are doing; none trigger interventions that spare one from the untoward consequences of the particular disease with any meaningful likelihood. Screening is not a bad idea; these are just bad screening tests.

This would not come as a surprise to the public-health establishment were it not so blinded by (and heavily subsidized for) their zeal to find disease early and smite it a mighty blow. They all should have been exposed to Bayesian statistics in their training. In order to find a condition in a population that is largely spared that condition, you need a very good test. The less frequent the condition, the more the test must approach perfect. For example, let's say you have a very precise test for condition X, a test that is 98 percent sensitive and 98 percent specific. The sensitivity means that if you have 100 people with condition X, the test will be positive in 98 of them (a 2 percent false-negative rate). The specificity means that if you have 100 people who do not have the disease, the test will be positive in only two of them (a 2 percent false-positive rate). That's a pretty good test. Let's say you screen a general population where only one person in 1,000 has X (that's a highly prevalent condition). You have a meager chance of finding that one person, but for every one you find, you'll declare at least nineteen positive who don't have the disease.

Screening is even more daunting since this hypothetical assumed a very precise test, meaning that it actually measures something very accurately and reproducibly. Most screening tests are not nearly so precise. Some, such as mammography, are operator dependent, so that different radiologists see different shadows differently. So, too, with colonoscopy and sigmoidoscopy; different endoscopists can find or miss cancers in any particular patient. Some tests, such as cholesterol, PSA, and HbA1C, are measuring normal constituents in blood and defining "abnormal" by consensus based on consideration of the range of values in various populations. The cutoff is never a clean divide. These tests are doomed to result in many false positives and many false negatives. If you're going to advise screening, you have to be certain that the result is not a lot of unnecessary harm and that whatever harm is meted out to some is easily justified by the good done to others.

As I said above and have said before, many sanctioned screening tests are bad tests for the purpose of screening. Some of these same tests are much better as diagnostic tests—tests used to seek the cause of a relevant symptom, which increases the prior probability that the patient has the disease in the first place. Because they are sanctioned as screening tests by august bodies, they have a life of their own, particularly in America. Submitting to them is accepted as a sign of health literacy by most Americans. Furthermore, screening is promulgated by an enormous and enormously profitable multifaceted enterprise. I suspect all will remain part of American "health" until they are superseded by the next generation of screening tests. Many on the horizon are as inherently flawed as these. Some are already in practice, such as the "screening" tests foisted on elderly people who are concerned they have "mild cognitive impairment."

However, there are ways to design screening tests that do not repeat the mistakes of the fathers. One way forward is now on the cutting edge of the molecular biology revolution, absorbing the efforts of a great many scientists and the coffers of many a venture-capital fund. This approach is hidden in the proviso that I offered regarding screening for colorectal cancer: "without a family history of early life colorectal cancer." This sort of family history suggests a genetic predisposition. If we knew the gene(s) that predispose to colorectal cancer, we could screen only the carriers in the family with frequent colonoscopies starting early in life. It may turn out that the gene(s) are necessary for them to develop early cancer, but not sufficient; there may be other factors at play. That means some of the carriers are actually at no risk, but we cannot distinguish these from those destined to develop colorectal cancer. So all carriers in the family turn their sunny sides up annually from age forty or earlier.

Similar considerations pertain to women with the BRCA-1 and BRCA-2 genes. If a woman has one of these genes and also has a close relative who developed breast or ovarian cancer at an early age, her risk is substantial. Given the inadequacies of screening mammography even for this high-risk woman, most would advise her to undergo bilateral mastectomies. This is a horrifying undertaking for these young women, even if they are offered the rigors of breast reconstruction. Furthermore, it does not address their risk of ovarian cancer, where screening is useless and prophylactic surgery causes infertility. This is the state of the art for women with this genotype who have an afflicted close relative. But it is not the case for women with this genotype who do not have any relevant family history. Studies are under way to define their risk more precisely, but if it is increased at all, it is not dramatically increased. For example, about 2.5 percent of Israeli women have this genotype as opposed to about 0.25 percent of American women, yet the incidence of breast cancer is not elevated in Israel. As a result, there is no mandate to screen women for this genotype in the absence of the family history. The genes are necessary but not sufficient for dramatically increased risk, and "risk reduction" involves horrifying surgery rather than the unpleasantness of colonoscopy for colorectal cancer. BRCA-1 and BRCA-2 are genes that confer risk when something else about the woman's biology synergizes—a second hit. We don't know what that means mechanistically. Does it mean there are other genes yet to be identified that have products that enhance the malevolence of BRCA? Or are there influences that are not coded for in DNA itself that do the dirty deed? Both possibilities have well-studied precedents.

The implications for human genetics are considerable, even when single genes are not affording susceptibility but are directly responsible for a disease. Many such gene mutations are lethal. Many are fully penetrant, meaning that if you have the gene, you have the disease, such as with some forms of muscular dystrophy and of hemophilia. But many are far less predictable. Some are highly varied in the age of onset of disease and therefore of symptoms. This is the case with Huntington's chorea and hemochromatosis. Both of these diseases can be ascribed to mutations of one gene. We know the gene for each and could easily screen for it. There is a telling literature exploring the ethical conundrum of screening family members for Huntington's chorea. Would you want to know, since there's nothing we can do to prevent the onset of the brain degeneration? Would you want to go through life under the darker cloud of uncertainty as to *when* rather than the cloud as to *whether*?

There is also an ethical dilemma of screening for hemochromatosis. This is a disorder of iron metabolism in which iron slowly accumulates in the body, causing damage to liver, heart, pancreas, skin, and joints. We have several effective treatments, including simply removing a pint of blood from the patient with a frequency that keeps the iron stores reasonable. If there is a family history of the disease, we can screen family members for the gene and follow carriers with a simple blood test that monitors iron stores. The disease is seldom manifest in women before menopause, but it can sneak up on men much earlier. The conundrum relates to whether we should screen for this disease in the absence of a family history. Primary hemochromatosis is the commonest genetic disease in America, with one out of every 200–300 people carrying one copy of the high-risk C282Y genotype. Only four in 1,000 carry two copies and are at even greater risk. But there is tremendous variability in the age of onset and the severity of the disease, so that the vast majority of people with the genotype stay entirely well. There's the conundrum. The U.S. Preventive Services Task Force (*Annals of Internal Medicine* 145 [2006]: 204–8) feels that in the absence of a family history, a screening program cannot be recommended, even though about 6 percent of the individuals identified by screening already have some liver damage. This is the same august body that continues to recommend mammography in women older than fifty-five and younger than seventy with a far-more-tenuous rationale. Maybe they'd feel differently if there was a hemochromatosis advocacy movement that commandeered the public's attention with out-cries about rationing.

Genomics, Proteomics, and Statistics

There are many heritable traits, including behavioral traits. Some are favorable and hence termed "normal" if not fortunate; others are un-favorable and likely to qualify as "diseases" in the minds of too many. Nearly all of these traits are polygenic, meaning there is not a single, not even a predominate, gene whose gene product is the proximate cause of the trait. Rather, a particular array of genes and their products con-spires to create the biology that underlies what we call a genetic trait. The genes, single gene or polygenic, contributing to any trait are termed the genotype of the trait. As with single genes, the biology that can be as-cribed directly to the gene products is seldom manifest as the trait with-out first being exposed to environmental influences, including forces outside the body that perturb the internal cellular environment. These external forces range from bits of information leading to "learning" to the toxic petrochemical moieties we discussed above. The result of the inter-action between gene products and biological modification is what we see or measure as the phenotype. It is possible in some systems to measure the degree to which a particular phenotype is a product of the genotype, a measure termed heritability.

I am taking you through this terminology to provide you with weapons to place the media's zeal for medical genetics into perspective. Americans have come to speak, fear, exalt in, and banter about genetics. In her bril-liant and prescient monograph *Experiencing the New Genetics* (2000), an-thropologist Kaja Finkler discussed how "genetics" was already medical-izing the modern notions of family and kinship twenty years ago. Today, most people think they are stained if Uncle Bill died of a heart attack at seventy, and most think they are blessed if Uncle Jim lived to ninety-five. These people are wrong. There are genetic influences on the develop-ment of coronary artery disease and on longevity, but they are so slight as to be clinically irrelevant. These are barely heritable traits, despite all the hype and assumptions peppering the pronouncements in the media.

Not all polygenic traits are barely heritable. The onset and progression of degenerative changes in the spine, hands, and knees are largely heri-table; the influence of such environmental factors as usage is trivial in comparison. Performance on standardized tests of intellectual function is substantially, though far from entirely, heritable. So, too, is the likelihood of developing type 1 diabetes or ankylosing spondylitis. Most diseases are not at all heritable, though there are surprises. Susceptibility to tuberculosis is importantly heritable, though the intensity of exposure to the infecting bacteria can overwhelm whatever resistance to infection one inherits. However, chronic diseases like rheumatoid arthritis, systemic lupus erythematosus, type 2 diabetes, and many others have minor genetic components. This doesn't mean that the genetically determined biology, however minor, is irrelevant. Understanding these basic mechanisms may someday yield molecular secrets that can be harnessed to benefit patients. I am not one of the many critics of this theme in the science of genomics. However, I can see no advantage to knowing your own profile of susceptibilities at this stage of the science. What do you do with information such as you are 2 percent more likely than average to develop rheumatoid arthritis but 3 percent less likely than average to develop coronary artery disease? You can buy such information today, and companies are lining up to market to you tomorrow. You are forewarned.

Another theme in genomics is pharmacogenetics. Its goal is to identify genetic traits that influence drug metabolism. There are many examples of drugs that are metabolized more quickly in some people, even some ethnic groups, than in others. Alcohol is metabolized on average differently in Japanese people than in Caucasians. Genetically determined differences in the metabolism of pharmaceuticals have long been appreciated, but usually these differences are overcome by tailoring doses and dosing schedules to achieve efficacy without toxicity whether a particular patient metabolizes the drug slowly or quickly. Some of these circumstances have been studied to identify the genetic basis for enhanced or decreased susceptibility, such as the gene that predicts sensitivity to a drug used to treat the hepatitis C virus.

The Holy Grail for pharmacogenomics is in developing tumor-specific chemotherapeutic agents. We have very few effective chemotherapeutic treatments for cancer in general and for solid tumors in particular. Cancerous cells always have genotypic differences from the tissue they arose from, or they wouldn't be cancers. Furthermore, cancers arising from the same tissue in different patients often differ one from the other. Could it be that hidden in all this heterogeneity are particular genotypes that are susceptible to particular drugs but are missed because the susceptible tumors are only a fraction of the tumors from different patients? Of course this could be the case. There are laboratories dotting the landscape of molecular biology plowing these fields.

Such work is a frustrating exercise, as you would predict; there are minor differences in genotype, difficulties in demonstrating that any "gene signature" correlates with prognosis, difficult assays for drug susceptibility in the laboratory, and even greater challenges in testing therapeutic inferences at the bedside. Nonetheless, there are claims of success. One test for susceptibility to a chemotherapeutic agent, Oncotype DX, is marketed widely for breast cancer without compelling scientific support for its utility (such a study is under way, with funding from the National Cancer Institute). There are precedents for false starts, such as the Ova-Sure test, a proteomics test to detect early ovarian cancer developed by Professor Gil Mor at Yale that was licensed by the university and used on patients before it was shown to be useless. Proteomics is a method that parallels genomics; instead of looking for "gene signatures," it assays myriad proteins and protein fragments in blood looking for distributions that associate with clinical states and status. The statistical challenges are similarly immense, perhaps insurmountable.

I have little optimism that cancer pharmacogenomics will ever prove as successful as its proponents avow. The tests are based on assaying dozens of genes for over- or underexpression to develop the "gene signature" that might characterize a particular tumor. Then the investigators look at the clinical course of the patient with the particular tumor, seeking associations with drug susceptibility or with clinical features like the proclivity to metastasize. When they find associations, they are tenuous because of the tremendous variability of the assays and the clinical courses. In fact, there is a danger of repeatedly probing the data sets until one is fooled by an association that is nothing more than a statistical fluke. For that reason, no association can be relied on until it is tested prospectively in a separate group of patients. This is all so daunting, with pitfalls waiting at every turn. However, at the very least and before promise is trumpeted, these patients deserve the most rigorous of science. As David Ransohoff said in an editorial in *Nature* in 2005, "As new '-omics' fields are explored to assess molecular markers for cancer, bias will increasingly be recognized as the most important 'threat to validity' that must be addressed in the design, conduct, and interpretation of such research."

This is a field that is still prone to place the methods of molecular biology ahead of rigorous statistics needed to properly determine whether the inferences derived in the laboratory can advantage patients. It is also a field scarred by scandal. Some of it is a product of zeal and trashy science. Some of it is turning out to be worse than that. There is much at stake for patients, but also for scientists and their backers. Duke University is reeling from a scandal that arose when it turned out that its medical center was harboring and nurturing a scientist, Dr. Anil Potti, who had lied about his credentials and gone on to publish a series of "gene signatures" in lung cancers, purporting them to be therapeutic milestones with data that convinced his colleagues, oversight committees, funding agencies, and patients. He was found out when statisticians from the M.D. Anderson Cancer Center determined that his results could not be derived from his data. Caveat emptor.

The Forest and the Trees

No doubt we will make advances in avoiding diseases and in treating the diseases we didn't manage to avoid. But we will all die, nonetheless. Far more important than changing, even choosing, the disease that proves our reaper is gaining assurances that we do not die before our time and that our journey to our ripe old age was pleasing. In the modern world in resource-advantaged countries, promoting the latter is the overriding public-health mandate. Despite the din of the bells and whistles of the molecular biology community and the harsh, strident pronouncements of the environmental scientists, the only sensible approach to serving this mandate is to listen to the whispering of the disaffected, the disallowed, and the disavowed among us. The evidence-based recourse that begs our attention suggests we need to provide a welcoming community and a nurturing ecosystem.

The Department of Housing and Urban Development (HUD) heard the whispering and decided to test the suggestion. From 1994 to 1998, HUD undertook an extraordinary social experiment. Some 4,500 women with children living in public housing in highly disadvantaged urban settings were randomly assigned to one of three groups. One group received a housing voucher that could be redeemed only if they moved to a more-advantaged neighborhood, in which case they were afforded counseling to assist in the transition. A second group received the voucher without the counseling. The third group was left to their own devices.

It is too early to know with certainty whether this social engineering will afford important health advantages, but preliminary data suggest a very modest reduction in some of the relevant biological markers of health risk, such as morbid obesity and diabetes ("Neighborhoods, Obesity, and Diabetes: A Randomized Social Experiment," *New England Journal of Medicine* 365 [2011]: 1509–19). The experiment may prove as disappointing as the "Negative Income Tax" experiment undertaken during the Nixon administration. This involved randomizing disadvantaged families to various levels of income and counseling support. Even the group afforded the most made little progress in entering the mainstream of society ("A Comparison of Labor Supply Findings from Four Negative Income Tax Experiments," *Journal of Human Resources* 20 [1985]: 567–82). Maybe all the insights about the relationships between social capital and social cohesiveness and longevity are missing the forest—or maybe money with or without counseling is no match for inadequacies in these contextual attributes. We need a more inventive experiment that tests the salutary nature of inclusiveness. The disadvantaged who are afforded inclusivity will still die, but they will meet that fate at the same ripe old age as the advantaged in their birth cohort and with a sense of fulfillment. I'll toast that journey.

6

The Social Construction
of Health

I am unabashedly advocating the randomized controlled trial (RCT) as the foundation for the delivery of rational health care in the twenty-first century. If an intervention has been shown to offer a meaningful advantage to a group of patients in an RCT, it should be licensed for prescription in that group of patients. It should serve as the standard for comparison in comparative-effectiveness trials with whatever else is available or comes along for similar indications in other groups of patients. Until a meaningful benefit can be demonstrated in an RCT in a particular group of patients, the intervention should not be licensed. Furthermore, without the availability of an intervention with demonstrated efficacy, comparative-effectiveness trials are fatuous. This is the creed of evidence-based medicine.

This is a hard line to maintain, particularly since I am the first to admit that many a clinically important question has yet to be tested scientifically, and many more do not lend themselves to scientific testing because of the marvelous range of individual differences, the variability of our species, and challenges in defining and measuring outcomes. In these circumstances, there remains a pivotal role for astute observations, wisdom, common sense, and perspective. But this pivotal role must always be recognized as resting on the shakiness of inferential reasoning. Instead of fixed beliefs and intransigent argument, the next observation must be viewed as potentially more astute and as calling into question the prior wisdom, common sense, and perspective. This is a dialectic that is intrinsically conflictual. But enlightenment is to realize that controversy is the mother's milk of new knowledge. In this chapter, we will explore the blurry lines of demarcation between enlightening controversy and metaphysical arguments. I cannot sharpen the lines, but I can offer insights as to when one has overstepped into the realm of unsubstantiated belief.

Is the RCT the only incontrovertible way to test clinical hypotheses? Wouldn't observational data—observing patients' responses to therapy—alone serve in some circumstances? Certainly if there seems to be no efficacy in observational data, one would argue that there is little reason to go forward with an RCT. How about if there's dramatic efficacy? For example, imagine a cancer that is known to be uniformly fatal in six months. You have designed and synthesized a novel drug that in theory should work, one that seems very effective in an animal model of the disease and that's well tolerated in Phase I trials on normal volunteers. Now your Institutional Review Board (IRB) agrees it is ready for a Phase II trial in a small group of these desperate patients. After you fully inform them of your rationale and infuse them with your optimism, the patients volunteer. Six months later, only half are dead, and some of the remainder appear to be free of the disease. Isn't that compelling evidence that you have happened upon a eureka drug? Wouldn't further study of the agent in an RCT be superfluous, even unethical?

Maybe.

There are several ways you can be fooled by observational data of this nature. Two in particular are likely to hoodwink you into arguing for the wide prescription of your eureka drug when in fact it is far less efficacious than you think.

You are basing your dire prognosis on past experience. That's called a historical control or historical reference. But diseases have natural histories. For example, a sixty-year-old well man is 30 percent less likely to experience a heart attack today than his father was when his father was sixty. Furthermore, the five-year survival following a heart attack was 50 percent for the father but is 96 percent for the son. Almost none of this good news can be ascribed to anything but the shift in natural history. Diseases have dramatic natural histories. The death rate from tuberculosis and the incidence of rheumatic fever were rapidly declining long before we had specific antibiotics. Bubonic plague became less of a plague in the Middle Ages long before relevant improvements in hygiene were instituted. You wouldn't know that the "dire prognosis" of this hypothetical cancer was spontaneously improving if your point of reference was a generation ago; you can only learn that by setting up a contemporaneous control group. Otherwise, you'd be fooled into exalting your eureka drug, which may be far less efficacious, even useless.

Cancer is often staged on the basis of how far it has progressed. The more it has progressed—in particular, the more it has spread away from its primary site (metastasized)—the worse off you are and the more likely you are to die in the near term. The degree of spread is usually determined by imaging techniques. The techniques available a generation ago were relatively blunt. Tools like regular X-rays can only detect larger metastases in particular anatomical sites. So "early spread" a generation ago meant that overt metastases were detected while smaller metastases in other sites were missed. Today we can detect the smaller metastases with CT scans and MRIS (and PET to gild the lily). Today we can stage the cancer more accurately. If we compare today's treatment of early metastatic cancer with the treatment of "early metastatic disease" of the same cancer a generation ago, it will look like today's treatment is more efficacious because the patients live longer despite early metastatic disease. But this is a spurious inference. What was defined as early spread a generation ago is defined as more-advanced disease today. Likewise, "no metastatic disease" a generation ago has yielded to newer technologies that detect metastases much sooner. So yesterday's early disease is today's widely disseminated disease. This is called stage migration, and it is commonplace in the cancer chemotherapy literature with a time course measured in years, not generations. If stage migration is confounding the hypothetical Phase II trial we're discussing, the survivors at six months would have survived six months without the drug, and they may all be dead at a year as a reflection of the natural history of their disease. The late Alvan Feinstein, a pioneering Yale epidemiologist, called stage migration the "Will Rogers Effect" after the humorist's observation that when the "Okies" left Oklahoma for California, they raised the mean IQ of both states.

So it is possible to use observational data instead of RCTS to define efficacy, but valid inferences are very often elusive, even when there is a "hard" outcome such as the time between diagnosis and death or cure of many diseases. The challenges for designing RCTS are magnified greatly when the outcome is "soft," but the pitfalls to drawing valid inferences from observations of soft outcomes are nearly insurmountable.

Relieving Symptoms

Death is death. Cure is cure. But pain is not pain. Happiness is not happiness. Nor are many other symptoms, which vary greatly depending on who is suffering, who is observing, and why and when. It is not possible to rely solely on observational data to define efficacy when the outcome is soft. The experience is highly dependent on the psychosocial context in which the symptom is experienced, and its reporting is highly individualized. That means that the symptom that is recorded as an outcome in any study is highly dependent upon the degree to which the instrument used to elicit, record, and monitor the symptom is specific for and sensitive to the contextual and temporal variables. These methodological challenges can be unanticipated curve balls that hide within any observational data set. For example, the idiom "pain in the neck" is primarily used as an aspersion by native Mexicans in Mexico, whereas it is more likely to be a personal symptom when used by an American regardless of ethnicity. A similarly designed study of an intervention for neck pain north and south of the Mexican border will be comparing apples with pears unless these cultural differences are taken into account. This issue is far more general than this example. There is no reason to assume the course of the illness experience is the same in all contexts.

This is not to belittle an individual's response to the query, "Are you better?" The affirmative is the object of any course of treatment that any individual seeks out. It is also the goal of every therapeutic exercise. It is possible to seek out and elicit this response for no scientifically valid apparent reason. It just happened. Of course, "it just happened" is seldom sufficient to suppress the urge to guess at the reason. Such idiosyncratic events are commonplace in all treatment acts, as we will discuss shortly. But to scientifically test the best guess demands a definition of the population to be treated, a standardization of the treatment, and a valid, reliable measurement of the outcome—a measurement that is sensitive to meaningful improvement. This is also true when the outcome to be measured is "hard," like death or a heart attack, but it is daunting when the outcome to be measured in a treated population is a symptom for which there is no "hard" corollary. The outcome is perceptual. The outcome is subjective. The outcome is in the mind of the patient. Furthermore, the outcome is convincing to the mind of the observer.

Designing the measurement instrument requires understanding which aspect of the psychology of recalling or reporting any symptom is of interest. Take the example of low back pain. This symptom is a frequent intermittent predicament of life. We know from studies of people in the community that most do not report an episode, nor will they remember it for long. Some seek medical care. Some find the episode a cause of work incapacity that they can overcome. Others experience short- or long-term disability. While the pain in the back may be similar, in each circumstance the illness it provokes is quite different, both in manifestation and duration. For some, it is transient and memorable; for others, it is transient and not memorable; for still others, it overwhelms function. In the case of low back pain, there is a highly informative science dissecting these contingencies (see *Stabbed in the Back*). Any intervention for low back pain would have to be studied with methods appropriate to the context in which low back pain is suffered by the subjects in the study. An outcome such as "return to work" is very different from "feel better."

Placebo

Deciding which illness one wishes to study and what outcome is important is only the first hurdle in studying interventions for soft outcomes. Soft outcomes always vary over time. Furthermore, the temporal variation can reflect a change in the intensity of the symptom itself or a change in coping. How do you know your patient or any group of patients was about to do poorly or about to do better without your intervening? There are efforts to find predictive biological markers, but none has proved a match. The only way to deal with this variability is an RCT that randomizes subjects in the hopes that the tendency to spontaneous waxing and waning will distribute evenly. Studying soft outcomes is challenging for clinical investigators and very risky for pharmaceutical firms. The reason is that many subjects in the referent group, usually a placebo control group, are likely to do well. If the placebo-controlled group does well, the drug being studied fares poorly.

That's why there is a push for trials that compare two active drugs; since it is likely that the new drug will do as well as the old and there is some small chance it will do better, the new drug is at lesser risk of being found useless. This is why I call for a halt to such active-active trials unless we have compelling data that the old drug really works. Most trials of this nature need to be controlled by a treatment arm that is given an inert intervention—a placebo—or no intervention at all.

The history of placebo-controlled RCTs for soft outcomes is daunting, instructive, and remarkably recent. There is the famous experiment that

Benjamin Franklin performed at the behest of King Louis XVI in 1784 to debunk Franz Anton Mesmer's claim to curing all sorts of ailments with a healing principle he termed "animal magnetism." Franklin demonstrated that mesmerism was a salve for the symptoms of the gullible, causing Mesmer to set up shop in Switzerland. Mesmerism was not so easily banished; it thrived well into Victorian times and manages the occasional resurgence in the guise of various sorts of magnetic therapies up to the present.

The modern era of the placebo was ushered in by Henry Beecher. While a medical officer in World War II, Beecher observed that soldiers with dire wounds requested less pain medicine and made such requests surprisingly less often than soldiers with minor afflictions. Clearly, the experience of painfulness was subject to modification as a function of context and expectations. Beecher famously made this point in a 1955 paper titled "The Powerful Placebo" in the *Journal of the American Medical Society* (vol. 159, no. 17 [1955]: 1602–6) in which he reviewed his experiments and those of others on treating postoperative pain, headache, and other painful conditions with opiates, nonsteroidal analgesics, or placebos.

With a series of inventive experiments, Beecher demonstrated that only about a third of subjects across a wide range of painful conditions responded to placebos consistently and exquisitely, whereas another third were consistent nonresponders. He was convinced that placebo reactors were not suffering from "imagined pain" since they were often those with actual wounds and not just those with no objective cause of pain, such as in the case of headache. He realized that the reactors were those whose pain was accompanied by the "severest anxiety states." Nonetheless, he was convinced that the placebo can have a "powerful therapeutic effect." He noted that a significant percentage of patients treated with placebos suffer adverse events, usually symptoms that mimic those they would anticipate from opiates (somnolence, dry mouth, nausea, weakness, etc.). Beecher also realized that it was insufficient to just "blind" the subject in RCTs of the treatment of painful states. Such trials had to be "double-blind": neither the patient nor the monitoring investigator should be able to discern whether the treatment is the active drug or the placebo. The attitude of the investigator was a treatment act, just as the drug or placebo under study was a treatment.

Henry Beecher is one of the giants of twentieth-century medicine. He moved the clinical study of pain and its treatment to the forefront of clinical science. I was privileged to attend his lectures at the Massachusetts General Hospital when I was a third-year student at Harvard Medical

School in 1966. He was an engaging, imposing figure with an even-more-imposing intellect. At that late stage in his career, just before he retired as the founding chair of the Department of Anesthesiology, his focus was on defining the ethical constraints on clinical research (another of his great achievements). But he discussed his work on the placebo, which was still ongoing in his department. I vividly recall sitting in the gallery of an operating room watching a surgeon treat the extensive burn wounds a young woman had suffered. She was implacably passive through a procedure that is uniformly extraordinarily painful. The sole anesthetic was acupuncture. I saw the young woman again when I was a student on the psychiatry service. She had a major thought disorder, schizophrenia, which was a far-more-likely explanation for the implacable passivity than any putative effect of acupuncture. The anesthesiologists missed that point. They missed the critical nature of "double-blind" in their early work, too. None of Beecher's inferences about the "powerful therapeutic effect" of the placebo has withstood unscathed the science that followed. Neither is any totally discarded.

The Placebo-Controlled Double-Blind RCT

In studies with "soft" outcomes, the subjects given a placebo in an RCT usually do quite well. Sometimes they do as well as the subjects given the "active" drug, in which case the "active" drug is abandoned. Sometimes they do nearly as well, but rather than abandon the drug, the Contract Research Organization (CRO) or the sponsoring pharmaceutical firm usually reverts to a comparison with a similar licensed drug, an active-active comparison, in an experiment designed to allow for an assertion of noninferiority. Then the argument for licensure is based on some small advantage in convenience or toxicity. For symptomatic drugs that are licensed, the advantage over placebo is often anything but impressive, let alone compelling. Here are several examples:

- As we've discussed, most trials in cardiovascular medicine and surgery do not rely on hard outcomes, such as death from a heart attack or even a heart attack. They rely on soft outcomes, such as the frequency of exercise-induced angina (chest pain). Drugs to treat angina have fallen by the wayside in the mindset of the interventional cardiologists. They'd rather do angioplasties and bypass grafts. But many of these drugs were introduced and studied in RCTs. All that are licensed are more efficacious than placebo, but not by much. Whether the end point is pain running on a treadmill or frequency of angina going forward, all licensed drugs decrease the incidence by nearly 50 percent— but all placebo-treated patients in these trials did nearly as well at nearly 50 percent. The difference is statistically significant, or the FDA would not have been swayed to licensure. The FDA has licensed many pharmaceuticals for soft outcomes because a small increment in efficacy has been demonstrated in RCTs. This was a focus of an earlier chapter. Our focus in this chapter is the large minority of subjects in RCTs in many different clinical settings who are served as well by swallowing a sugar pill.

■ In *Rethinking Aging*, I detail the two RCTs on treating elderly women with acute, persistently painful osteoporotic compression fractures by injecting cement into the damaged part of the spine. In these RCTs, the placebo control was a sham injection. About a third of patients were dramatically better after either cement or sham injections despite having suffered for many months up to the intervention. This procedure has been covered by Medicare since 2001 based on the advice of the advisory panels on which the Centers for Medicare and Medicaid Services (CMS) relies. FDA approval was not necessary since the cement was long in use for other indications and the procedure itself required no novel device. By 2008 Medicare had paid for over 70,000 of these vertebroplasties at an average cost of $5,000 to $6,000 each.

Adam Elshaug and Alan Garber, prominent health-policy experts, rejoiced at the prospect of evidence driving considerable cost savings in an essay in the *New England Journal of Medicine* titled "How CER Could Pay for Itself: Insights from Vertebral Fracture Treatments" (vol. 364 [2011]: 1390–93). They did not foresee the aggressive and effective pushback that followed. In a paper in *Health Affairs*, Katherine Wulff and her colleagues at the Department of Bioethics in the National Institutes of Health discuss the unsuccessful attempt by the CMS to stop paying for a procedure that was no better than placebo in these trials ("Can Coverage Be Rescinded when Negative Trial Results Threaten a Popular Procedure? The Ongoing Saga of Vertebroplasty," *Health Affairs* 30 [2011]: 2269–76). The CMS yielded to political pressure by stakeholders whose arguments ranged from a criticism of the methodology to asserting that the study populations are not representative of the patient population that has responded in the past. The saga is an object lesson on how difficult it is to enforce evidence-based medicine after the fact, after any intervention is established in practice. Too much money and ego is invested in the status quo.

- In *Stabbed in the Back*, I detail myriad RCTs that relate to medical, alternative, and surgical interventions for regional low back pain. The control always does nearly as well, if not equally well, as the active intervention. Particularly in terms of a measure of painfulness, patients in both the active and the placebo limbs of trials tend to do quite well. If the outcome measure relates to return to work, claimants do comparably poorly regardless of the treatment.

- Life offers up many psychological challenges, times when sadness, anxiety, grief, and more are a pall. These are situational challenges that differ from spontaneous, inexplicable affective disorders now termed "major depressive disease." The situational challenges are not diseases, and successfully coping with or overcoming these challenges is a definition of health. But they are intermittent and ubiquitous challenges that whet the appetite of the pharmaceutical industry and for which many a pill has been marketed, expected by patients, and prescribed. All are licensed because of RCTs that demonstrate improvement in both the active drug and placebo limbs, a little more in the active limb. However, the difference is small in the licensing trials and does not replicate over time. Jonah Lehrer's essay in the *New Yorker*, "The Truth Wears Off" (December 13, 2010), does more justice to this observation than the purveyance of psychotropic agents to treat life's predicaments does for patients.

The fact that so many subjects in so many soft-outcome RCTs do well on placebo has not escaped notice. For decades, the phenomenon was dismissed as a demonstration of the "natural history" of the illness under study. That interpretation applies to "hard" outcomes such as kidney function and the like. If an RCT is testing whether an agent improves kidney function, any improvement in the placebo group must temper the estimate of any positive drug effect observed in the patients on the active drug. But "natural history" is not an adequate explanation for any improvement in symptoms observed in the placebo group.

Symptoms tend to wax and wane in all circumstances, but the "placebo response" demonstrated in an RCT is never merely a reflection of the tendency toward spontaneously waning. Both the act of volunteering and the fact of participating distort the "natural history." One can assume that the "placebo response" affected the illness experience whether the subject received the placebo or the active drug. The RCT is asking whether the active drug is producing enough of a specific health effect that its addition to the placebo effect is discernible.

One is left to ponder how much simply participating in the trial is therapeutic. This quantity is elusive. Any attempt to do less than administer a placebo designed to be indistinguishable from the active agent borders on an active-active trial design, and doing nothing (usual care or some such) can be a biased comparator given the ethical constraints on recruiting subjects to RCTs. Subjects are subjects because their consent is "informed." If the placebo treatment is familiar and ordinary, can you expect a placebo effect? If you tell someone how to recognize the placebo in an RCT, is it still a placebo? The answers are not as straightforward as one might think at first blush. Before we explore them, there are other aspects of the RCT that need wider recognition. Nothing about this topic is straightforward.

The Placebo-Controlled Double-Blind RCT in the New Age

In theory, an RCT recruits subjects that are representative of the population with the affliction and then randomly assigns them to active and control treatments without introducing bias. That means neither the subject nor the observer can know whether the subject is receiving the active intervention or the control. This can work perfectly in an RCT where the subjects are inbred mice. Clinical investigations always violate these parameters, and they always should. First, subjects are recruited from accessible populations by offering inducements. The accessibility may reflect institutional affiliations, peer networks of the principal investigators, targets of some sort of public advertising, or, often, all of these. The inducements may include stated or implied hope/expectation of benefit, gratis medical care, financial remuneration, or combinations of such. As a result, it is likely that the volunteer population is not representative of the entire afflicted population. To the contrary, there are "stables" of volunteers that tend to volunteer repeatedly for particular conditions. Furthermore, since the "stables" are limited in number and the demand for volunteers seemingly limitless, new "stables" are popping up all over, including in Africa, Asia, and South America.

All volunteers for trials carry preconceptions and expectations that may differ from those of patients with the same disease undergoing treatment in clinical rather than research settings. In the clinical setting, rational treatment should depend on informed medical decision making. In the research setting, the treatment is driven by possibility and inducement rather than by established precedent. In the research setting, the preconceptions and the expectations inform the volunteering, but the decision to treat is co-opted by randomization. The research volunteer cannot choose the treatment; the patient should.

To enter the study, the volunteer must offer "informed consent." This is a stylized interaction that involves the signing of a detailed consent form, the content of which has been approved by an institutional review board. The principal investigator or a designee is to read the form with the volunteer and explain any portion that is confusing. In a previous chapter, we used the example of a consent form for angioplasty to illustrate the fashion in which consent forms for interventions assume the likelihood of benefit and emphasize the possibility of adverse events.

Consent forms for RCTs emphasize the possibility of benefit and the likelihood of adverse events. Ethicists like Steven Joffe of the Dana Farber Institute and Jeffrey Peppercorn of Duke University have dissected the conundrum of presenting benefit-risk information in a fashion that sacrifices neither the best interests of the volunteer who seeks personal benefit nor those of society at large, for which a negative outcome is almost as valuable as a positive one. For me, the ethical conundrum can be obviated whenever the aim of the RCT is to discern a small effect, as is true of many trials, particularly in cancer chemotherapy. The patient is far less likely to become a subject if such were explained. Would you volunteer for an RCT if you were informed that if you are randomized to the active limb, you are at substantial risk of a litany of adverse effects, and the most benefit you can hope for is a few extra months of longevity? Seldom, if ever, is the volunteer offered such a realistic estimate of the potential for benefit. I feel strongly that glossing over this aspect in the consent process is unethical. Such a trial should not be done.

But I digress. We are not considering the RCT with hard outcomes like longevity. We are considering the information that one presents to the volunteer so that he or she might consent to participate in an RCT with a soft outcome without prejudicing that outcome. This is less of a challenge if the active agent is itself totally anonymous, such as a tasteless, odorless pill one takes at home. Then the preconceptions of the volunteers operate similarly whether they are randomized to the active agent or an equally anonymous placebo pill. If the active agent is not anonymous, preconceived notions of efficacy can color the response. That bias can be unavoidable and insurmountable, as in trials of zinc-containing potions to thwart the common cold. All such potions have a distinctive taste because of the zinc. There is no way to know if the subject feels better in anticipation of the efficacy of the distinctive-tasting potion or because the potion somehow enhances the body's response to viral upper respiratory infections.

When the active intervention is unmistakable, designing the trial is particularly challenging. This is the rule for RCTs where a physical modality is studied, such as acupuncture or some form of manipulation. Subjects volunteer because something in the procurement is enticing. In all likelihood, the naming of the active intervention caught their attention and the description of the active intervention during the consenting process had some degree of appeal. Otherwise, they are less likely to volunteer or consent or persist in one or the other limb of the trial. This mindset predisposes to improvement in soft outcomes; everyone anticipates benefit, including those who are physically applying the active intervention to the subject's body. These interventionalists need to be secure in their skillfulness, which usually means a belief in its benefits. The subject and the person applying the "modality" are both likely to magnify change in that direction.

Hence, it behooves the investigator to contrive a comparison intervention that might be viewed by the volunteers (yes, they speak to each other) as better than a default. "Usual care" and less-frequent personal contact with the investigators are convenient comparators but not a fair test of the efficacy of the active intervention. Even exquisitely designed sham modalities can fail if the operator seems less enthusiastic. Perhaps one can avoid overt bias in an RCT if the modality is a machine that is applied to the body (a transcutaneous electrical nerve stimulation [TENS] unit or a diathermy machine) where the volunteer can't tell if the machine is turned on or not. In fact, many such studies have been done for back pain and similar illnesses, and it doesn't matter whether the machine is turned on. There have also been many studies comparing various forms of spinal manipulation with each other, with other modalities, and with usual care for regional low back pain. If the volunteers are recruited from a young population that is naïve to all forms of laying on of hands and has no issues relating to work incapacity, there is a small but reproducible benefit from a single, simple osteopathic back crack compared to laying on of hands without cracking. Otherwise the likelihood of added benefit from spinal manipulation in RCTs correlates with the belief of the volunteer at the time of consent that the manipulation will help. The more skeptical the volunteer, the less likely he will be pleased by the outcome.

One of the most elegant demonstrations of this was a study from the Brigham Hospital in Boston published in the *British Medical Journal* in 2006 (doi: 10.1136/bmj.38726.603310.55). It was an RCT for persistent arm pain in 270 subjects. Actually, there were two simultaneous RCTs. In one, half the volunteers were randomized to receive the drug amitriptyline or a placebo pill every day. In the other, they were randomized to acupuncture or sham acupuncture. The acupuncture was performed twice weekly by an experienced acupuncturist in a standard traditional fashion, except that the fine needles were sheathed. In the sham acupuncture, the sheathed needle was placed in a standard location but the needle was not advanced into the skin; in the active group, it was advanced into the skin. The subjects were not able to discern the difference in technique. The genius of this study is that it was not undertaken to compare active treatments with placebo controls. The study was designed to compare the two controls—sham acupuncture and a sugar pill. Over the course of six weeks, there was a decrease in arm pain in subjects whether they were exposed to the sham acupuncture or the sugar pill, but the decrease was greater and sooner in response to sham acupuncture. Interestingly, 15 percent of the subjects receiving sham acupuncture experienced pain during treatment, and 10 percent noticed an increase in pain after the needle was "removed."

Sectarian Medicine

As I said, explaining away the placebo effect as simply a fortuitous swing in the natural history of the illness is reasonable when the outcome is hard, but for a soft outcome—symptoms—it is naïve. Clearly, preconceptions of beneficence on the part of the patient enhanced by the belief in benefit by the person applying or offering the placebo play a major role. This is obvious if one reflects on the history of health care. It is a history of successive and coexisting therapeutic beliefs that have been the basis for distinctive systems of care that capture those for whom the beliefs resonate.

Some systems claimed a scientific basis so that the interventions could be couched in scientific jargon and unproved scientific hypotheses. As already mentioned, one example of the former that has not survived intact is mesmerism, an eighteenth-century vitalistic theory involving magnetism that exercised Benjamin Franklin to undertake a form of RCT, which sent Mesmer and his theory reeling. At about the same time, Samuel Hahnemann was formulating homeopathy, a system of care that will not fade into history even though it is based on scientific theories that have proved untenable. There are many similar systems where practitioners and adherents are unshaken by the fact that their "scientific" beliefs are either untenable after scientific testing or simply cannot be tested.

Truth be told, much that was purveyed by my guild, by "Doctors of Medicine," prior to World War II qualifies for this description, and much of common practice proved harmful when my guild's reliance on science became more than lip service. Today, physicians can look down on the other systems of care and label them "sectarian" because they lack a substantive evidentiary basis for their claims of benefit. My guild is wont to consider the claims of sectarian medicine as examples of how some people can be "fooled" by placebo effects.

The response of sectarian systems in twentieth-century America to this criticism has varied considerably. Osteopathy and the American branch of homeopathy allowed themselves to be largely absorbed into my guild. The chiropractic touts the scientific demonstration of a slight degree of benefit in one subset of their patients as validating their entire system of care. Some of the sectarian systems find no need to get embroiled in the science debate. These systems are comfortable with the metaphysical notions on which they base their care. This tradition is even more colorful and more successful than sectarian systems purporting a scientific basis; it is steeped in religion. All religions offer access to comforting. Some offer access to faith-based healing as a central tenet, such as Christian Science and the Pentecostal movement. All offer up anecdotes of therapeutic triumph, some of which are quite dramatic. If they mobilized scientific explanations and justifications, they too would be examples of sectarian medicine. But they don't bother with that.

Scientific medicine, sectarian medicine, and metaphysical belief systems have one thing in common: all offer comfort and comforting for those who seek them out. And all who seek them out share the particular therapeutic beliefs with the particular purveyors and providers. There was a time, before World War II, when the choosing was laissez-faire. It no longer is. If anyone is faced with the possibility of a damaging underlying disease, it is irrational if not criminal to exclude scientific medicine from recourse. Prayers, spinal manipulation, homeopathic remedies, and what have you are no match for my guild in treating serious bacterial infections, abdominal and obstetrical catastrophes, some tumors, some inflammatory diseases, and much more. Modernity demands that you check out the advantages of evidence-based medicine before, or even while, seeking comfort in whatever fashion you find comforting. And that includes religion.

If you're fortunate, you can find a physician who laces evidence-based medicine with comforting. Such has been an ideal for centuries. It was the prescription of Francis Bacon (1561–1626) in his Essay XXX, *Of Regimen of Health*:

> Physicians are some of them so pleasing and comfortable to the humour of the patient, as they press not the true cure of the disease; and some other are so regular in proceeding according to art for the disease, as they respect not sufficiently for the condition of the patient.
>
> Take one of a middle temper; or, if it not be found in one man, combine two of either sort; and forget not to call as well the best acquainted with your body, as the best reputed of for his faculty.

Faith Healing

There are strident critics of organized religions. Some of the most articulate are avowed atheists who argue that organized religion lacks redeeming features. The polemics of Christopher Hitchens in *God Is Not Great* and *The Portable Atheist* (both 2007) and of Richard Dawkins in *The God Delusion* (2006) are influential and extreme examples of the arguments that denigrate all metaphysical thinking. I am far more moderate and tolerant in my personal philosophy. I stated as much publicly when I offered my voice in defense of the nomination of Francis Collins, M.D., Ph.D., to be director of the National Institutes of Health (http://www .healthbeatblog.com/2009/07/dr-nortin-m-hadler-tells-all-you-need -to-know-about-the-new-head-of-the-nih.html). Francis was the pioneering molecular geneticist who directed the Human Genome Project. Long before that, he was a medical student at the University of North Carolina, entering with a Ph.D. in physics from Yale. During his student years, he became a devout Christian, and in 2006 he expressed his philosophy in *The Language of God: A Scientist Presents Evidence for Belief.* There was great opposition to his appointment in part because of his religious beliefs.

Francis Collins was one of the first medical students to teach me the joy of mentoring and the reward of watching a student flourish when I was a very junior faculty member at the UNC School of Medicine in the 1970s. There have been many others over the years, including Francis Collins's daughter a generation later. Francis harnessed his particular genius to create an extraordinarily distinguished career. His contributions to our understanding of human genetics speak for themselves. But that is the least of his genius. Francis understood and explained the fashion in which these scientific "advances" are incremental rather than revelatory. Francis understood and explained how these "advances" can have ramifications that are harmful if not recognized and discussed openly. Francis understood and explained why science is an exercise in refutation; no one should presume the result of the experiment yet to be done. In a society that has been taught that money can purchase a cure for every physical and emotional disorder, Francis is a beacon of enlightenment.

Francis also understands how little we really know. He is not the first scientist to come to that realization; to the contrary, it is an inescapable conclusion. Some, including myself, live comfortably with uncertainty. Others, including Francis, need an explanation, even if the explanation is beyond testing. As a geneticist, Francis argues that the common goodness of human beings is evidence for a higher power. I respect this argument, and I value the fact that he can readily countenance my doubts about the robustness of the evidence for common goodness and my lack of comfort with a metaphysical explanation.

To the degree that faith in any metaphysical system of beliefs offers comfort to an adherent who is ill, faith has value in any health-care system. Some, such as Harold Koenig of Duke University's Center for Spirituality, Theology, and Health, try valiantly to generate some scientific underpinning for a salutary effect of faith beyond palliation. Koenig's book *Medicine, Religion and Health: Where Science and Spirituality Meet* (2008) is testimony to his convictions. But there is no way to design an unbiased RCT of the health benefits of a religious belief system. Belief is too idiosyncratic. There is also no easy way to quantify any adverse effects in this particular regard. These, too, are highly individualized. The polemics of a Hitchens or a Dawkins relate to blights of religion on societies more than on individuals, blights that result from xenophobia and competing theological and economic agendas. But if someone who is ill finds a degree of comfort in religious ideation, I see no reason to do anything but acknowledge the mindset. If there are no claims for "cure," only for relief from suffering, and the "modality" doesn't challenge my notions of acceptable (as in exorcism, *limpieza de sangre*, or the like) and there is no coercion, then the ill person has chosen to participate in an "I believe you can help me" palliative event. From my perspective, it qualifies as a placebo event, but palliative nonetheless.

Placebos as Deception

I mentioned that while my guild, Doctors of Medicine, has always claimed stake to the summit of "scientific reasoning," it is only since World War II that it has generated an evidentiary basis for such a claim. The Citizen Patient is learning to recognize when and where modern "scientific medicine" deserves to strut in this fashion. However, there are elements of the modern medical treatment act that are and will always be based on mutual beliefs. Much of the substance of chapter 8 discusses the aspects of the "clinic" that qualify as such. There is a chapter in *Stabbed in the Back* where I discuss sectarian medicine in detail because so many belief systems have related to notions of "spine" and its disorders. However, the subtitle of that chapter is "My Name is Nortin and I'm a Placebo?" because I discuss the palliative aspect of the notion of "bedside manner."

The mind is a wonderful thing that clearly can be fooled, and fooled with, so as to perceive something that is anticipated whenever the preconception is reinforced by the strength of the personality and personal convictions of the treating agent. From studies like the sham acupuncture study, it is clear that the mind can be fooled even in the absence of the force of personality in the treatment act. The science purporting that placebo effects can alter the progression of destructive disease processes is a will-o'-the-wisp. But the science demonstrating the fashion in which symptoms can be ameliorated by placebos is not so readily dismissed. That is also the conclusion of Asbjørn Hróbjartsson and Peter Gøtzsche of the Nordic Cochrane Centre writing for the Cochrane Collaboration.* They have reviewed the relevant literature repeatedly over the years and last came to this conclusion in a review published in issue 1 of the Cochrane Library in 2010 (doi: 10.1002/14651858.DC003974.pub3). The conclusion is based on a systematic review of over 200 RCTs on sixty

---

* This is an organization based in Oxford, UK, and funded by contributions from multiple federal governments. It now has thousands of scientists assembled into over fifty Review Groups, each responsible for formulating questions on a particular clinical topic, reviewing the relevant clinical literature, grading the literature as to its methodological quality, and attempting to deduce an answer to the question that is weighted toward the studies deemed highest in quality. The resulting documents, already approaching 10,000 in number, are published, collected, frequently updated, and made readily accessible.

different clinical conditions. All were designed to compare some putatively "active" intervention with no special treatment. For example, in a trial in asthmatic patients published in the *New England Journal of Medicine*, both the placebo and the no-treatment groups were still afforded customary care for asthma ("Active Albuterol or Placebo, Sham Acupuncture, or No Intervention in Asthma," *New England Journal of Medicine* 365 [2011]: 119–26). There was no difference in measured lung function, but the placebo treated group felt less breathless.

In all RCTs comparing placebo interventions with no special treatment, the subjects are told the placebo is an active intervention. Would anyone volunteer if they were told the study was designed to test the efficacy of a modality believed to be a placebo? If they volunteered, would they be prejudiced to find the placebo useless? Fortunately, some highly inventive investigators are applying themselves to the study of placebo effects, investigators who are not cowed by the counterintuitive. These are investigators like Ted Kaptchuk at the Osher Research Center at Harvard Medical School and Franklin Miller of the Department of Bioethics at the National Institutes of Health. The two often collaborate, merging their unusual backgrounds and often adding others from as far afield as semiotics. Kaptchuk earned a doctorate of Oriental medicine from the Macao Institute of Chinese Medicine in China. Frank Miller holds a Ph.D. in philosophy from Columbia University and specializes in bioethics. These two and their collaborators undertook an RCT of prescribing a placebo in a small group of volunteers with irritable bowel syndrome (IBS) recruited by advertising a study for a "novel mind-body management." The trial compares no special treatment with telling the patients to take "placebo pills made of an inert substance, like sugar pills, that have been shown in clinical studies to produce significant improvement in IBS symptoms through mind-body self-healing processes." The principal result is presented in Figure 6.

IBS is one of a family of disorders characterized by persistent and intense symptoms in the absence of any important demonstrable underlying disease. We will have more to say about these disorders shortly. IBS is diagnosed when diarrhea, constipation, and abdominal pain are the principal symptoms in any order or combination. The patients randomized to taking pills were given a bottle clearly labeled "placebo pills . . . take 2 pills twice daily." The primary outcome of the four outcomes illustrated in Figure 6 is the "Global Improvement Score," which asks whether the symptoms over the past week have (1) been substantially worse, (2) been moderately worse, (3) been slightly worse, (4) undergone

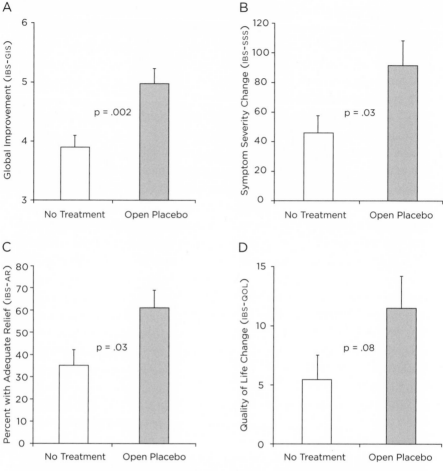

Figure 6. Results at two weeks of an RCT comparing a treatment offered as a "placebo" with no special treatment in patients with irritable bowel syndrome. This is a figure from the original paper published by T. J. Kaptchuk and others, "Placebos without Deception: A Randomized Controlled Trial in Irritable Bowel Syndrome," *PLoS ONE* 5, no. 12 (2010): e15591; doi: 10.1371/journal.pone.0015591. The result in panel C is particularly noteworthy. Nearly 60 percent of the subjects on placebo experienced "adequate relief" at two weeks. This is much more than the 30 to 40 percent generally seen in the placebo limb of pharmaceutical trials. (A. Hróbjartsson, P. C. Gøtzsche, "Placebo Interventions for All Clinical Conditions," Cochrane Database of Systematic Reviews 1 (2010): CD003974; doi: 10.1002/14651858.CD003974.pub3)

no change, (5) slightly improved, (6) moderately improved, or (7) substantially improved. The symptoms of those patients who were not given placebo pills stayed about the same. However, those who took placebo pills did a bit better. The fact that 60 percent claimed adequate relief at two weeks is an even-more-impressive statistic.

It is hard to escape the conclusion that the combination of the attitude of the investigators and the "mind-body" rationale overwhelmed whatever might be dissuasive in knowing that they were swallowing a placebo. The claim by the authors that they were able to demonstrate the effect of placebo without deceiving the subjects about being on a placebo begs reflection, however. The claim is based on the belief that the mind-body rationale is what Michel Foucault would term an *épisteme*, a fundamental ground state of knowledge. I disagree. I will argue that mind-body is a semiotic, symbolic of notions held dear by these subjects that are anything but epistemic. This is not simply an abstruse argument played out with philosophical jargon. If I am correct and mind-body symbolizes something very different, even magical to these subjects, then they are as much deceived by mind-body as if they had been told the placebo pill was an active agent.

Nocebo

Placebo is Latin for "I will please." Nocebo is Latin for "I will harm." Both terms were introduced into the medical lexicon in the early 1960s, in the early days of pharmaceutical RCTs. Placebo has made its way into parlance. Nocebo remains more obscure, and I have no need to see it otherwise. But it denotes a phenomenon that deserves close scrutiny. Despite all good intentions, might a placebo cause harm? Is it possible that something that you believe to be totally benign and should be completely inert turns out to be a nocebo? For example, there might be a trace of a substance in your placebo pill to which a rare individual is violently allergic. But that's not why I'm bothering you with the nocebo notion.

Revisit Figure 6. There is another explanation for the slight but statistically significant difference in outcome between the subjects who swallowed the placebo pill and those who didn't. Both groups had volunteered for the study, understood its design, and participated in the same therapeutic/investigative milieu populated by individuals who evinced concern, empathy, and attention. One would predict that symptoms would be alleviated by such a treatment environment, and indeed, both groups improved. Perhaps the greater improvement seen in the group swallowing the pills is what one would expect if this treatment environment could be replicated without the study. Perhaps the group afforded usual care in the study resented being deprived of pills said to open the path to "mind-body self-healing processes." This resentment or disappointment could very well blunt the advantages the other group derived by virtue of diving head first into this particular clinical milieu. If this were true, the mind-body pill is the placebo and the control exposure was a nocebo. This possibility is as consistent with the data in Figure 6 as is the prior explanation that seemed so sensible.

When we discussed sectarian medicine, I pointed out that each of the various disciplines wields their form of intervention, a "modality," with conviction bolstered by theory that is usually dressed up in scientific garb. All the practitioners and professionals, licensed or otherwise, who offer to push you, pull you, poke you, gird your loins, ply you with potions, alter your diet, and so much more have their theories. Many of these theories have been put to the test in RCTs. The results are generally inconsistent; whenever efficacy is demonstrated, it's slight. Nearly all the modality RCTs have methodological flaws, often flaws that cannot be totally circumvented given the difficulties in designing scientifically adequate control treatments. After all, most modalities are much more than a technique; they invoke interpersonal relationships and expectations. Without some expectation of benefit, subjects are less likely to experience benefit. The closer the experimental design comes to isolating the modality, the less likely one is to observe any hint of efficacy.

That's why my guild is wont to call all this "sectarian medicine." As Norman Gevitz asserts in *Other Healers* (1988), the rubric denotes "organized movements seeking professional status" for the purveyance of placebos to people who expect them to salve their symptoms. It is true that the patients of sectarian practitioners have a great tendency to return again and again for the same illness or its recurrence. Sectarian medicine mobilizes a plethora of testimonials from their patients in response to the criticisms of my guild. Nonetheless, society has decided to elevate many forms of sectarian medicine into the realms of the acceptable, the advisable, and even the indemnifiable. Advocates and purveyors are at least as visible today as their forebears were a century ago, although the menu of modalities and theories has changed. Around the mid-twentieth century, there was something of a hiatus, but it was fleeting.

There is no doubt that all of these testimonials are a reflection of the degree to which patients who participate in sectarian medicine feel better after becoming involved in these treatment acts. Are we as sure that these people are better off for feeling better in this fashion? All sectarian treatment acts are instructional; the patient/client learns the jargon and accepts the theory. Most go through life with a view of their health that is altered to conform to this new line of reasoning. Many can sample more than one form of sectarian medicine and somehow incorporate more than one line of reasoning, although seldom do so simultaneously; they switch lanes when they see the need. Medical anthropologists term this "medical pluralism."

These patients feel better for these efforts, but have they become well? Many a medical philosopher has tried to come to grips with a definition of health, a gold standard to satisfy this query. My definition incorporates an element of invincibility, the sense that nothing can happen to me that I can't cope with. There are patients of mine with destructive inflammatory diseases like rheumatoid arthritis or lupus who manage to be "well" by this standard. There is a wealth of data demonstrating that patients who participate in sectarian medical systems seldom are well. They view themselves as having whatever theoretical flaw they learned they have, they have a good deal of anticipatory anxiety, and they have a tendency to catastrophize. No wonder they are quick to return for persistence of symptoms and any hint of recurrence. To the extent this pertains to any given patient, sectarian medicine is a nocebo.

My guild is not without blame in this context. It is a residuum of a paternalistic tradition. Educators like me argue that the role of the physician is to turn patients back into people, even if they are people coping with chronic or fatal diseases for which treatment is guided by informed medical decision making and fostered by an ongoing relationship with the physician. This was one of the themes of my last book, *Rethinking Aging*. However, it is difficult if not impossible to discuss the distinction between my guild and sectarian medicine without inflaming passions. I am trying to be as evenhanded as I can. I draw a distinction between my guild, the institution of medicine, and medical professionalism. I am not gentle about the former, while I remain idealistic about the latter. I use the term "guild" advisedly. I am aware that the self-serving monopolistic posture of medieval craft guilds was not viable in an open market.

Much Ado about Nothing

The tendency for discussions of sectarian medicine to trend toward the inflammatory, even toward the invective, is as old as the competing guilds and professions. It played out between organized medicine and the chiropractic in the twentieth century. Before 1983 the ethical code of the American Medical Association stated that it was unethical for a medical doctor to associate with an "unscientific practitioner." The AMA's Committee on Quackery labeled the chiropractic an "unscientific cult." Needless to say, there was no love lost between the respective professional organizations. One result was a lawsuit under the Sherman Antitrust Act brought by Chester A. Wilk, D.C., and several colleagues in 1976. They lost the first suit and appealed. The decision in the appeal did not satisfy either party, so both appealed. In 1990 the U.S. Court of Appeals for the 7th Circuit found in favor of the chiropractors (895 F.2d 352) because "the AMA failed to establish that throughout the relevant period [1966–1980] their [the AMA's] concern for scientific methods in patient care had been objectively reasonable." The U.S. Supreme Court has refused, repeatedly, to revisit this case, as it involves no novel point of law. There's still no love lost between the professions, though I am free and willing to accept referrals from chiropractors.

Most of the debates, discussions, and vitriol between sectarian groups and between these groups and my profession play out in the court of public opinion. One might think this would be less true in the twenty-first century thanks to the intercalation of an informative science into the debate over the meaning and value of the placebo. Maybe that will happen, but there's little sign of it yet. Even the leading academic investigators can be embroiled. Some, like Kaptchuk, have managed to stay largely above the fray. He has gained sufficient professional credibility to garner a faculty position at Harvard without a recognized doctoral degree and has sufficient clout to warrant being featured in a *New Yorker* magazine essay titled "The Power of Nothing" (December 12, 2011). Ted Kaptchuk and Franklin Miller maintain a scientific perspective in their writings, even to the extent that they can coauthor a paper titled "Placebo Effect Studies Are Susceptible to Response Bias and to Other Types of Biases" with Asbjørn Hróbjartsson, the Danish investigator whose Cochrane Review found little that would nurture the advocates for some special therapeutic value of placebos (doi: 10.1016/j.jclinepi.2011.01.008).

Other investigators have not avoided stepping in a bear trap. Edzard Ernst was recruited from his chair in physical medicine and rehabilitation at the University of Vienna to be the professor of complementary medicine at Britain's Peninsula College of Medicine when it was founded in 2000. Ernst was the first professor of complementary medicine anywhere. He is now retired but still quite visible and prolific. He was recruited because he was comfortable with, and a practitioner of, a number of the therapeutic modalities that were eschewed by mainstream medicine, homeopathy in particular. He set out to design studies that would provide scientific substantiation for approaches that are grouped under the complementary-medicine rubric. Over the next nearly two decades, he published some thirty RCTs, the book *Trick or Treatment: Alternative Medicine on Trial* (2008), and literally hundreds of reviews, many of which are systematic analyses of the literature. As professor of complementary medicine, he became one of its most prolific, strident, and visible critics. This culminated in a public brouhaha in 2011 when Ernst accused Prince Charles of being a "snake-oil" salesman. Prince Charles is an advocate for complementary and alternative medicine. Furthermore, Prince Charles created the Foundation for Integrated Health, which apparently purveys such potions as a "detox remedy" made from dandelions and artichokes. Both the *British Medical Journal* (doi: 10.1136/bmj.d4937) and *The Guardian* newspaper (July 29, 2011) have covered the resulting colorful (if nothing else) feud. Ernst argues his creed in a 2011 editorial in *Rheumatology* (doi: 10.1093/rheumatology/keq265): "The recognition of the therapeutic value of an empathic consultation is by no means a new insight, yet it is knowledge that is in danger of being forgotten . . . (by) mainstream medicine . . . where alternative practitioners tend to provide the non-specific and mainstream doctors the specific effects."

Placebo effects, their purveyors, and the attendant theoretical baggage have both wide appeal and extraordinary staying power, at least as much today as at any time in the past. Society at large tends to gloss over reductionistic critiques such as mine, Ernst's, and the Cochrane Review, while adherents to placebo-based health-care systems tend to consider them personal insults and are resentful. More surprising is the general ignorance of the rationale for evidence-based medicine. Kristin Carman and her colleagues at the American Institutes for Research, a CRO for behavioral research, published a survey demonstrating that most people do not want to let evidence shake their beliefs ("Evidence That Consumers Are Skeptical about Evidence-Based Health Care," *Health Affairs* 29 [2010]: 1400–1406). With this as "common sense," placebo-based therapies cannot cause cognitive dissonance; the more the merrier.

Mind-Body Duality

Today's theoretical baggage is as vitalistic as it was a century ago, when everyone seemed comfortable with the postulates invoking all sorts of special bodily forces. Today, the postulates involve the latest invocation of the "mind-body" paradigm. We entered the twenty-first century wedded to the belief that "It's in your mind" is an imprecation—akin to accusing you of imagining something, in this case some symptom, or even of fabricating the symptom. It is customary to anchor such thinking in the writings and teaching of René Descartes (1596–1650). Descartes was fascinated by the phenomenon of the phantom limb, the observation that an amputee is likely to experience sensations in an amputated appendage. It was in this context that he wrote that "nature likewise teaches me by these sensations of pain, hunger, thirst . . . that I am not only lodged in my body as a pilot in a vessel, but that I am besides so intimately conjoined . . . that my mind and body compose a certain unity." (*Meditations on First Philosophy*). Descartes put cognition in the brain and emotion in the "mind." To my way of thinking, the Cartesian mind-body paradigm foreshadowed the work of George Engel at the University of Rochester during the last century. Engel formulated the "biopsychosocial" model of illness that underlies much of my writing. The illness experience is a consequence of the interactions of cognitive cerebral processing of inputs from the ravages of disease and the psychosocial context in which it is suffered. In this model, all illness experience is "in your mind," regardless of the underlying disease. I've written for years that I want one American patient to go to an American physician and say, "Doc, I feel awful—could it be in my mind?," and have the physician respond: "I hope so. That's much better than leukemia or renal failure or lots else." To this day, such a chief complaint is anathema.

It's not anathema as a Cartesian legacy. The legacy derives from another debate that occupied many philosophers and theologians in the seventeenth century. That debate was about "soul." Soul was beyond or above "mind," but where and what was it? If one name is to be associated with the idea that "in your mind" is an imprecation, I'd offer up a contemporary of Descartes, Blaise Pascal (1623–62), who stood in strong opposition to the rationalism of Descartes. Pascal was recognized for his mathematical genius by age fourteen and had made indelible contributions to analytic geometry by his late twenties. At age thirty-one, following a road accident that he barely survived, he abandoned mathematics for theology and the teachings of Jansenism, a Christian theosophy that was considered heresy by the Roman Catholic Church. Pascal had suffered mightily from multiple somatic symptoms from childhood on, symptoms that he and his contemporaries described in detail. Pascal came to believe that it was natural and necessary for man to suffer, that the "ills of the body are nothing more than punishment for the ills of the soul." I spent a sabbatical as a visiting professor at Hôpital Cochin in Paris, a rambling institution in the middle of which are the remains of the Port Royal monastery, the center of the Jansenite movement to which Pascal retired for the last years of his life. It has a beautiful cloister, sheltered from the hubbub of the city and the hospital. You could imagine this ill, irritable, devout, frail young man walking this courtyard and composing *Pensées*. For over 300 years, we have been contending with notions of mind and soul and body that incorporated the sinister elements Pascal left behind when he took to his early grave.

Today, the rationalism of Descartes is assuming primacy. We're not ready for "It's in your mind," but we're getting closer. We're so close that Kaptchuk and his colleagues (Figure 6) could entice patients with irritable bowel syndrome to swallow "placebo pills made of an inert substance, like sugar pills, that have been shown in clinical studies to produce significant improvement in IBS symptoms through mind-body self-healing processes." There are several explanations for this transition of mind-body duality from mystical to acceptably modern. One is that the "biopsychosocial model" is widely accepted in medical circles. I'm not sure it is fully understood by the general public, but it *sounds* like it is legitimating mind-body duality and therefore is. This is a phenomenon termed "linguistic determinism." We can change concepts just by changing their name. If there is any doubt that mind-body duality is a modern, scientifically sound concept, it has been expunged by the rapid accumulation of a scientific literature demonstrating that the biology of the brain changes in response to lots of things, including emotions. To the public mind, this demonstrates with finality that "in your mind" is a biological construct, not something that one can be blamed for or should feel embarrassed by.

This is an overinterpretation of the science. There are neuroimaging techniques based on MRI and PET platforms that probe the regional metabolism of the brain and can do so dynamically. There are regions of the brain that "light up" with metabolic activity in response to many inputs, including emotions. The studies are difficult to do because the changes are subtle and not reliable, meaning they vary from subject to subject and over time in a single subject. Nonetheless, they are an advance in our understanding of how the brain functions. We've known for generations that different parts of the brain serve different categories of function, such as skin sensation, movement, and emotions. Now we can see the metabolic activation of these different parts when they are functioning. We've known that there must be fine differences between people

in the wiring in different brain regions that accounts for differences between people. But functional neuroimaging is no match for such fine detail. We know that wiring must change when we learn something new or
forget something. We even have animal models of such changing; Eric
Kandel deserved his 2000 Nobel Prize for sorting out the way the wiring
of sea slugs accounts for their behavioral changes. But the difference in
the complexity of the human brain compared to sea slugs is more than
night and day. And functional neuroimaging does not come close to the
resolution necessary to understand individual differences at any but the
crudest level. It is an advance, but to move these results into the clinical
arena is molecular phrenology. All that is accomplished is to allow people
to talk about mind-body processes and swallow mind-body placebo pills.

Medicalizing Misery

It has also given impetus to a second tidal wave of medicalization. The first
we have already discussed; that's where life's ubiquitous predicaments
like backache and grief are considered diseases to be treated with the
mindset one brings to the treatment of pneumonia. We know these to be
predicaments of life thanks to a generation of epidemiologists who ventured forth into the community and asked people, "How goes it?" Most of
this work would focus on a particular predicament: knee pain, foot pain,
bowel symptoms, headache, and the like. We learned how many and how
often people experienced such symptoms and dealt with them as people.
Nearly all of these folks considered themselves to be basically well even
though something important was coloring their day. Only a small percentage felt compelled to seek medical care. One of the pioneering community epidemiologists, Lois Verbrugge, termed this an "iceberg of morbidity": only a small fraction of people were at the tip, where they were
patients and likely to be medicalized.

More recently, community epidemiology has been less restrictive in
the probing. Epidemiologists began to ask people what else was going
on. Depending on how they ask the question, at any given moment, some
5 percent of the population is coping with more than one symptom. They
have all sorts of combinations of symptoms at the same time or sequen-
tially. And they have a lot else in common. They tend to consider themselves unwell despite the fact that nearly all of them have no definable
underlying disease. They are vigilant in terms of bodily symptoms and
tend to assume that the next is likely to represent a severe disease. The
vigilance causes anticipatory anxiety, and the assumption of severity is

termed catastrophizing. In fact, they are no more likely to suffer any of the diseases they fear than similar people who consider themselves basically well. Nonetheless, they will die sooner than others in their birth cohort who consider themselves well, die sooner of something (all-cause mortality) rather than simply be at risk for a particular disease. They are a bit more likely to suffer with depression than others in their birth cohort, but most don't. They are also more likely to be disadvantaged in terms of education, income, and job satisfaction.

These people live life under a pall. They visit physicians and other health-care providers frequently. Multiple diagnostic evaluations prove disappointing to a patient who is increasingly desperate for the definition of the cause of his or her misery. As was true of the epidemiologists who missed this forest for the trees, primary-care physicians tend to latch on to one aspect or another of the illness narrative when referring these folks on to the next level of diagnostic exercise. All physicians for generations have been aware of this patient population. Most do not greet such a patient's entry into the clinic with pleasing anticipation. These tend to be "difficult" patients who are usually dealt with by prescribing symptomatic relief during brief contact.

The illness experience of these unfortunate people is diffuse, persistent, and manifold. It plays out against a cultural system that superimposes expectations of "abnormal" on the narrative of illness. Idioms of distress are elicited to conform to societal expectations and to diagnostic preconceptions. So if the component of the illness experience that is drawn to the fore is a bowel complaint, shouldn't the diagnosis reflect that component, even if there is no obvious abnormality in the bowel structure or physiology? Hence a label such as "irritable bowel syndrome" can serve the need of the patient and the clinician for "the diagnosis," with the expectation that a cure then becomes possible, even if it is possible only "someday." If achiness emerges as the prime component, the label is "fibromyalgia." If it's pervasive, persistent fatigue, it's "chronic fatigue syndrome." These are the Big Three—labels that denote a quality of illness experience in the absence of demonstrable explicatory disease. There are other labels focusing on symptoms, such as "seasonal affective disorder" or "restless leg syndrome." All of these labels have much in common aside from the absence of biological abnormality: they lend themselves to acronyms (IBS, CFS, FM, SAD, RLS, etc.), they foster advocacy groups, and they promulgate sectarian physicians who are so comfortable in this milieu that they claim expertise. For years, these experts and their patients circled the wagons against all in the mainstream who accused them codependence, mind games, placebo medicine, and the like. They unfurled theories and harnessed anger to validate their beliefs. What is clear is that the contract between the practitioners and their patients is cast in cement. The practitioners become intransigent, and their patients become far less likely to leave the sect than people with similar symptoms who never became patients of these experts. That observation is difficult to interpret; one could argue that the most severely afflicted are the most likely to end up entrenched in these practices.

All of this changed with the entry of what Kristin Barker termed "diagnostic entrepreneurs" in her book *The Fibromyalgia Story: Medical Authority and Women's Worlds of Pain* (2005). The acronyms became rallying cries for committees of sectarian practitioners who formulated criteria for each of the acronyms. All such criteria begin with the caveat that diagnostic studies seeking disorders of relevant organ systems are negative. There follows an attempt to quantify symptoms so that those who are labeled have more than others who are not so labeled. It's an exercise in circular reasoning at best. For many criteria, such as the many "tender points" that were said to be characteristic of fibromyalgia, the uniqueness of the criteria proved ephemeral when studied scientifically. Nonetheless, armed with criteria and bolstered by patients with influence, the acronyms moved into the sights of the general public and even into congressional statements of legitimacy.

More important, the pharmaceutical industry became cognizant of this potential market teeming with needy patients. Pharmaceutical entrepreneurs found that many a diagnostic entrepreneur was a willing partner. The FDA in its wisdom first allowed an inroad by offering to review the efficacy of drugs for fibromyalgia twenty years ago. The floodgates then opened, both in terms of RCTs and of the direct-to-consumer marketing of their findings concerning all the acronyms and other symptoms of unknown origin. Let's stick with the example of fibromyalgia as an object lesson in how a pervasive illness experience can be reframed as a disease worthy of aggressive empirical treatment.

Mongering Disease

It is not difficult to find advertising and marketing schemes devoted to this end. They are a staple diet for the health-promoting broadcast and print media. A prototype fibromyalgia "advertisement" is Pfizer Pharmaceutical's spread showing the profile of a young woman, face glowing but skull revealing a magenta image of her brain. No drug is mentioned;

the stated intent is to inform as to the "evolving view of a controversial condition." In bold print, the header announces: "Fibromyalgia: 'Neurotic' or Neurologic?" The text goes on to infer that the problem is the latter, that "pain is amplified" by "pain-processing areas of the brain." This header begs close attention. It offers as much insight into the way we think of health as it does into why Pfizer is attempting to program and influence that thinking. Why should any person, patient, physician, or pharmaceutical-marketing agency think we would consider "neurologic" better than, or even different from, "neurotic"?

"Neurosis" is an antiquated term, expunged from the psychiatric lexicon but not from parlance. Sigmund Freud and Carl Jung used the term to denote psychiatric illnesses in which anxiety-provoking emotional distress leads to physical and mental symptoms. These range from normal human experiences all the way to phobias, hysteria, and depression but not to disordered thought processes like schizophrenia. The notion and term subsequently became an accusation of weakness rather than an assertion that one's coping style needs correction. The current psychiatric terminology would label those with a neurosis manifested as physical symptomatology as having a "somatoform" disorder—a rubric that I find as confusing as neurosis and that most of the large number of sufferers find as insulting as "neurotic." Yet somatoform disorder is a commonly used medical and psychiatric diagnosis to denote the patients we've discussed who mix anticipatory anxiety and catastrophizing in coping with unpleasant bodily (somatic) sensations. To my way of thinking, they are suffering from a very bad idea, and they need to be taught a better idea (i.e., undergo "cognitive behavior therapy," in today's jargon). More important, anyone with a tendency toward such a bad idea needs to be forewarned and deserves to be offered alternatives in reasoning long before the bad idea becomes entrenched, an *idée fixe*, even an obsession.

The evidence for using the label of "neurologic disorder in pain amplification" is another exercise in circular reasoning, to my way of thinking. It is based on functional magnetic resonance imaging. Patients whose narrative of illness garnered the fibromyalgia label may produce an image that is distinctive, particularly when faced with a painful stimulus. The differences are subtle, not particularly reproducible or specific, and are readily affected by stimuli like having an empathic family member present. Furthermore, this subtle change in reactivity may be a learned consequence of life under a pall rather than a cause of the illness experience. The fibromyalgists, their patients, and the support groups are leaping to this new imaging as evidence for "disease." Their enthusiasm has substantial underwriting from the pharmaceutical firms Pfizer, Lilly, and the upstart Cypress Bioscience.

This is not the first time the pharmaceutical industry has tried to establish a foothold for the benefit of all the people faced with persistent physical symptoms of unknown cause. Merck tried to co-opt this market for Flexeril® (cyclobenzaprine), its first-generation tricyclic antidepressant, over twenty years ago. At the time, the drug was not touted as an antidepressant since the implication would be offensive to these patients. Rather, it was marketed as a muscle relaxant, which might be useful in "fibrositis." Fibrositis was the predecessor label for fibromyalgia. Furthermore, the notion of a "muscle relaxant" is fatuous on scientific grounds. In trying to educate all involved, Merck underwrote a symposium and, partially, the American Rheumatism Association Committee that crafted the now-discredited 1990 American College of Rheumatology Criteria for Fibromyalgia. Flexeril never captured FDA approval for this indication and never captured this market off-label; few patients persisted in taking an agent that made them groggier than they already perceived themselves to be. But the market potential is enormous, and the quest to serve it has never died. It is now coming to harvest in the form of several recently approved drugs for treating fibromyalgia.

In June 2007 Lyrica® (pregabalin) became the first drug ever to be licensed by the FDA specifically for the treatment of fibromyalgia. Pregabalin is one of many compounds in search of clinical utility resulting from the molecular biology revolution. This one alters calcium channels in nerve cells and seemed to have tranquilizing and anticonvulsant activity in animal models. Pfizer convinced the FDA that the drug had a role to play in the treatment of seizures and diabetic neuropathy, and then it convinced physicians to write about 600,000 prescriptions for these indications, with the average patient footing a monthly bill approaching $150.

The approval for fibromyalgia is a testimony to the mindset of the FDA when faced with the perseverance of Pfizer in sponsoring multiple trials with marginal if not disappointing results. In the first trial, published in 2005, there was less than a point improvement on a ten-point scale for pain, and this change was statistically significant only at the highest dose studied. However, "dizziness" and "somnolence" was the price paid by over half of the subjects exposed to this dose. Interestingly, only 10 percent of those on placebo experienced "dizziness" and 5 percent "somnolence." This makes me wonder how the effects were monitored, since "nonrestorative sleep" is nearly ubiquitous in the illness narrative of this patient population, and neurological symptoms such as lightheadedness are nearly as prevalent. How were half the subjects on pregabalin able to distinguish the adverse event of "somnolence," given their prevalence of nonrestorative sleep? It is therefore not surprising that licensing was withheld pending firmer evidence. This resulted in the "Freedom Trial." In this trial, 1,051 patients were treated with pregabalin for six weeks in escalating doses to determine a dose that was tolerated and seemingly effective. Of the 54 percent still on the drug at six weeks, 287 were randomized to placebo and 279 stayed on their tolerated and putatively effective pregabalin dose. More of those who were randomized to take a placebo relapsed in the withdrawal phase. I can't imagine that blinding was possible in this design, given the high likelihood of drug-related adverse events that would alert people as to whether they were getting the drug or the placebo. By the end of five months, a third of the patients still on placebo and two-thirds randomized to pregabalin had yet to revert to baseline symptoms. This convinced the FDA of the drug's efficacy, and licensure followed. Pfizer has been rewarded handsomely. The patients have not. That's an opinion shared by others who have reviewed these trials, such as Anne Siler and her colleagues in the American Pain Society's *Journal of Pain* (vol. 12 [April 2011]: 407–15). For those patients who tolerate the agent, the most striking effect is that it has further cemented their obsession with the need to "cure" their disease.

A year later, Cymbalta® (duloxetine) followed pregabalin as the second drug to be approved by the FDA specifically for fibromyalgia. Duloxetine is a drug that was already licensed for the treatment of depression and diabetic neuropathy. The theory underlying the use of duloxetine in fibromyalgia is contrived; in the trial, published in 2005, the rationale was that "central monoaminergic neurotransmission may play a role in its etiology." This leap was enough for Eli Lilly and Company to sponsor the several trials that led to licensure, after which the company embarked on an aggressive marketing campaign to sell the expensive drug. These trials have much in common with the pregabalin trials. Many patients (as many as half) dropped out of a trial early on. Of those who persisted, the difference in efficacy between drug and placebo over six months is underwhelming. There was about a 10 percent absolute difference in the many outcome measures purporting to assess pain and other components of the illness experience. Furthermore, this small difference occurred in the setting of considerable nuisance. In the duloxetine trials, nearly half of the subjects on the agent (versus less than 15 percent on placebo) tolerated nausea caused by the treatment. Duloxetine also has considerable potential for liver toxicity and a disconcerting tendency to predispose to suicidal ideation.

Milnacipran is a variation on the duloxetine theme that has been marketed for depression in Europe as Ixel° for the past decade. Cypress Bioscience bought the exclusive rights for approval and marketing of this drug in the United States and Canada in 2003 and partnered with Forest Pharmaceuticals in January 2006 to undertake a Phase III RCT. This multicenter trial involved 1,200 patients labeled with fibromyalgia. The results are similar to the other agents: one can barely discern a degree of benefit in the face of readily apparent adverse effects. Savella° was licensed on a wave of prelicensing marketing and has been a blockbuster for the manufacturers. In this case, one can spot a number of the diagnostic entrepreneurs on the advisory and other boards of Cypress. Many are involved in the RCTs and "educational" agendas that led to licensing and swarm to the call of post-licensure marketing. This is a very lucrative business.

I am impressed with the industry agenda—impressed by its tenacity in undertaking and underwriting so many trials, its use of composite outcomes and other examples of data massaging, and its recruitment of fellow-traveling rheumatologists. The same handful of names appears on the masthead of the papers reporting the trials regardless of the drug or sponsor; the list is always accompanied by revelatory statements concerning paid consultancies and board memberships. This is one happy, conspiratorial family trying to convince these sad patients that "it's in your mind" is a New Age disease requiring pharmaceutical intervention. And they are convincing many. Across the land, patients ask their doctors if fibromyalgia is the reason they feel so poorly. Across the land, doctors have been "detailed" about these drugs and have closets full of samples. Across the land, there are patients tolerating toxicities because of the belief that they have achieved a degree of relief that is not so obvious to anyone who knows them.

I realize that anyone bearing the fibromyalgia label finds this overview infuriating. It is not my intent to cause them anguish. Anger is counterproductive as a therapeutic event. I apologize, but I intend to forewarn anyone who is not yet labeled and thus cannot gloss over this example of disease mongering. These people deserve to be informed as to the basis for the label and the consequences of labeling before they find themselves in this vortex. Once labeled, it's difficult to feel well ever again. I'd urge all to read Susan Greenhalgh's *Under the Medical Gaze* (2001). This book and Kristen Barker's book cited above are scholarly treatises by academicians who offer up a wealth of useful insights using fibromyalgia as their focus. But this wealth of insights is highly relevant for many in all age groups who have difficulty coping with symptoms of unknown origin. No parent should allow their fretful infant to be labeled GERD or their difficult child ADD or Asperger's without demanding to be informed as to the basis and consequence. Likewise, no adult should accept a pre-dementia label for being worried about forgetfulness or start swallowing "antidepressants" for reactive depression without making an informed decision. And no Citizen Patient should accept any of the acronyms we've discussed without a thorough appreciation of their implications.

7

Extricating Health Care from the Perversities of Its Delivery System

It is no exaggeration to say that the United States' standing in the world depends on its success in constraining this health-care cost explosion; unless it does, the country will eventually face a severe fiscal crisis or a crippling inability to invest in other areas.
—*Peter R. Orszag*, Foreign Affairs *90, no. 4 (2011): 42–56*

Peter Orszag is a celebrated economist currently working in the upper echelons at Citigroup. He cut his teeth in realpolitik in the Clinton administration and resurfaced in Washington, first as the director of the Congressional Budget Office and then as director of the Office of Management and Budget in the Obama White House. Orszag, along with Harvard professor David Cutler, another brilliant retread from the Clinton administration, were intellectual drivers of the historic Affordable Care Act, the health-reform act passed by Congress in March 2010. "The new law," wrote Orszag in a 2011 article in *Foreign Affairs*, "set up health exchanges through which individuals can purchase insurance, required those without health insurance to buy it, and created subsidies to offset part of the cost of insurance, especially for moderate-income households. The bill also reduced payments from Medicare and Medicaid to providers, imposed a new tax on high-cost insurance plans and created a set of new institutions intended to bolster quality and reduce costs throughout the system. Even before it passed, the health act became mired in political controversy, and its future remains at risk." I have not had occasion to discuss health policy with Orszag. Cutler sought me out while he was serving as senior advisor on health for Senator Barack Obama during the 2008 presidential campaign. I suggested that the approach they were taking and that was embodied in the Affordable Care Act perpetuated all that was morally bankrupt about the American health-care system. Furthermore, as the fiscal remedy that was the Grail of their public policy, it was doomed. I argued that if "health care" could take the moral high ground, the nation would be rewarded with better health at a very tolerable cost. Reforming the "health-care system" before reforming health care was worse than futile. But economists are too engaged by the challenge of containing costs to wonder if they were buying a "pig in a poke" or evaluate the real costs of the system.

I am no stranger to the inner workings of the health and disability insurance systems and have known and even collaborated with leading labor and health econometricians throughout my career. I was elected to membership in the National Academy of Social Insurance for this aspect of my scholarship. Econometricians and actuaries are comfortable working with and reworking large observational data sets. They are most keen on outcomes that are monetary, or surrogate outcomes such as employment parameters. It is exceedingly difficult for econometricians to wrap their minds around the inadequacies in their categorizations. For example, the possibility that compensable back "injuries" are surrogate measures for job insecurity or job dissatisfaction is seldom factored into the calculations of labor economists. Furthermore, it is difficult for them to take into account the possibility that something in common use might be useless, something such as surgery for a back "injury." And if it's useless, I don't care how efficiently, well, or cheaply it's done—I don't want it done. I told Cutler that focusing on cost rather than on efficacy was putting the cart before the horse and doomed the effort. I was not surprised he could not hear me. There simply is too much entropy in the profitability of the status quo. Perhaps Citizen Patients can hear me now.

I have been reflecting on and writing about a health-care delivery system that put the horse of cost before the cart of efficacy for over a decade. It's time for an update, which follows, and which is nurtured by the observations and principles detailed in earlier chapters. Abraham Lincoln is said to have observed that you can fool some of the people all of the time and all of the people some of the time. Americans bear him out when it comes to their health-care system. But one can hardly blame them. There is so much smoke and so many mirrors, such a din of half truths and falsehoods, and so many threats of "it could be worse" that any change in the system seems to risk death from Damocles's sword, let alone "socialized medicine." So the American people are patsies for the self-interests of those who profit from the status quo. So, too, are our representatives in Washington and in every state capital where "health-industry" lobbyists swarm like locusts. Any proposal that is arguably or even compellingly rational is met with the imprecation "rationing" by those whose profits are at risk. Even discussions of compassion and perspective at the end of life elicits the denunciation "death panels" from those who profit from turning the last months of life into a technological/pharmacological gauntlet. The response of the "people" is to resort to the safe harbor of leaving well enough alone—if only they could. As Orszag argues, the economics of the status quo will sink America. I would add that the economics of the status quo will toss one family at a time overboard while America sinks.

Orszag's voice is just one in the choir and far from the shrillest. Decrying the American "health-care system" and any proposal for an alternative is itself an industry. Academics pick at it endlessly, politicians beat their chests, policy wonks are busy pitching concepts like quality and disparity, and employers are imposing management strategies on benefit programs that are more appropriate to other aspects of a private- or public-sector enterprise. Meanwhile, moral entrepreneurs are promoting "prevention strategies" and tests for risk factors that lead to no demonstrable clinical benefit. Rather, and paradoxically, the resulting medicalization tends to inflate costs. With or without overmedicalization, the American medical enterprise is primed to treat disease with interventions of questionable benefit offered with glossed-over risks and resulting in ludicrous costs. All the while, the print and broadcast media bombard us with an industry-supported cacophony of marketing masquerading as health advice.

The United States has constructed the most irrational health-care delivery system on the planet. So many entrepreneurs are doing well at the cost of so many patients being poorly served and so many people not served at all (Figure 7). In terms of health disparities, the industry is plagued by unconscionable benefit-cost ratios, expenditures that cripple the unsuspecting insured as well as the uninsured ill, and treatments that are more harmful than helpful. And the system is simply not economically supportable. This truth is far less evident to the American mind, which is taught to think only in the economic context. We spent over a trillion dollars in 2011, some 17 percent of our gross domestic product. That's

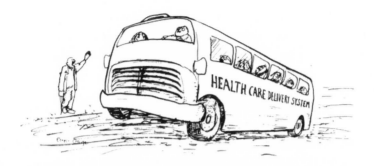

Figure 7. I was privileged to know the late Ernest Craige, M.D., as a friend and colleague on the faculty of the University of North Carolina for many decades. Ernie was a truly distinguished North Carolinian. He was the scion of a family that traced its roots in North Carolina to colonial times. His distinguished undergraduate career at UNC earned him a Rhodes Scholarship, after which he matriculated for an M.D. at Harvard and trained in medicine and cardiology at the Massachusetts General Hospital. He was one of several cardiologists to have been mentored by the legendary Paul Dudley White, and he carried the tradition of clinical acuity, compassion, and perspective with him throughout his life. Through the early decades of the twentieth century, the medical school of the University of North Carolina offered only the two-year preclinical curriculum, after which it sent its graduates to other institutions to complete the requirements for the M.D. degree. In the mid-1950s, the legislature of North Carolina decided to build the medical school into a four-year institution that granted an M.D. degree and to build North Carolina Memorial Hospital as its teaching hospital. Reece Berryhill was the founding dean. He set about the task of recruiting a clinical faculty and cleverly opted to find North Carolinians in the diaspora. Ernie Craige was enticed back home as the founding chief of cardiology. He was a legendary educator and an exemplary physician. He was a renowned clinical scientist instrumental in the development of echocardiography. He was also an excellent artist and a brilliant cartoonist. His cartoons found their way into many a medical publication, *Pharos* in particular.

For years, Ernie and I sat side by side at medical grand rounds. We whispered to each other about the content of presentations. Ernie was wont to turn to the blank side of the handout and draw cartoons about the theme of the presentation. Many were gifts to me. I have a collection that I cherish. This is one of his drawings. It captures the essence of the system we need to reform.

over twice the percentage of any other country, and for what? We stand dumbstruck when we realize that the "cost" of Medicare is rapidly escalating, and like sheep we tolerate the escalating pass-through of these costs. Most of this is painfully obvious to all of us, except maybe the overpricing. For example, for comparable drugs, the price per pill in the United States is 50 percent higher than in EU countries. In 2006 we were spending about $450 per capita to administer our system; no other country came close. France spent $250 per capita; Canada, $150; and Denmark, Finland, and South Korea were under $100 per capita. Administrative costs in the United States are prime examples of massaging data. So much that is unheard of elsewhere, such as the enormous advertising budgets of hospitals and clinics and the redundancies in "clinical staffing," is hidden in categories other than administration. For example, in the United States, the majority of in-patient nurses are supervisors who are not considered part of the administrative overhead since they are housed in proximity to the patients rather than in posh administrative towers.

I don't want to belabor this. The Orszags and the Cutlers are better equipped than I am—if they could learn to separate the wheat from the chaff. Besides, I believe that it is practically impossible now to dramatically alter the U.S. system; we missed the opportunity for a national health scheme in 1912 when it was a plank in the Bull Moose (Progressive) Party platform and a theme of Theodore Roosevelt's Bully Pulpit. Woodrow Wilson defeated Roosevelt and his Progressive platform. The best we can do today is impose rationality on the current system—ironclad, science-supported, and patient-driven rationality with the goal of assuring health and providing recourse when that assurance falls short. We are advantaged by a cadre of physicians who are culled from the ranks of the best and the brightest and who would like nothing better than to do what is right by their patients. America seldom hears of them, but rest assured that honest, caring physicians are out there in numbers.

And we are advantaged by lessons learned from the attempt to bring some rationality to the system undertaken by the Obama White House. As I said, arguing for rationality on the basis of cost will not solve the problem. The battle cry should be, "If it does not work, do not pay for it." That's not rationing. That's rational. That's the starting point. And if it does "work," how often does it work, and to what degree is it beneficial? The challenge is in defining efficacy in an entrepreneurial climate that gives no quarter. With efficacy as the first principle, defining the "common good" is an exercise in defining the shared values, ideals, and goals of the community. The agendas, values, and goals of purveyors, providers, and other "stakeholders" are rendered transparent.

The preceding chapters of *Citizen Patient* are written so that all Citizen Patients are primed for the climbing. I will reemphasize some of the guideposts as we ascend the trail.

Putting the Health-Care Cart in Front of the Health-Care Horse

In the debates regarding health-care reform, one goal promoted by all is "quality." If only we could perform up to standards, the institution of American medicine would be supreme and vindicated. Myocardial infarction provides a good test of this model, but eliciting "quality" in the treatment of heart attacks with carrots and sticks does not appear to improve outcome.* Those whose minds and mind-sets are fixed on improving quality argue that we must do what we are doing even better. I argue that what we are doing is useless at best and likely to be harmful. My argument is based on the literature that examines the effectiveness of what we do despite the theory, and the industry, that is committed to the current approach. The American approach to coronary artery disease is unsurpassed in terms of Type II Medical Malpractice, my term for doing the unnecessary even if it is done very well.

Quality of performance is not a goal in and of itself. It is only a goal if the performance benefits patients! Between Type II Medical Malpractice and excessive administration and profit, the majority of the "health-care dollar" expended in the United States does not benefit patients. So many high-ticket items that are trumpeted as the triumphs of U.S. medicine are little more than a scam. Spine surgery for regional low back pain, interventional cardiology/cardiovascular surgery for coronary artery disease, and arthroscopy have earned this ignominy. The first priority for reform in the care of the health of the American is to stop underwriting the profitably useless. We have the science to do so.

Evidence for Efficacy Underpins Evidence for Effectiveness

I discussed the difference between evidence for efficacy and evidence for effectiveness in chapter 3. Evidence for efficacy offers one some degree of confidence that a particular association, say between a drug and a good clinical outcome in a particular clinical setting, is not likely to have occurred by chance. Effectiveness asks the crucial next question: given any particular instance of efficacy, do you really care? Is the effect important enough, likely enough, and safe enough to be valuable to me? The science that informs utility hinges on this distinction between efficacy and effectiveness.

Efficacy explores whether something ever works; effectiveness explores whether it works well enough to matter in practice. The only com-

* There have been many attempts to demonstrate meaningful benefits that have largely disappointed the "quality" proponents. For example, see S. W. Glickman SW, F.-S. Ou, E. R. DeLong, M. T. Roe, B. L. Lytle, J. Mulgund, J. S. Rumsfeld, W. B. Gibler, E. M. Ohman, K. A. Schulman, and E. D. Peterson, "Pay for Performance, Quality of Care and Outcomes in Acute Myocardial Infarction," *Journal of the American Medical Association* 297 (2007): 2373–80.

pelling evidence for clinical efficacy, for an association between an exposure (a drug or device, for example) and a health effect, comes from randomized controlled trials. Every other scientific research design is more susceptible to confounding, bias, and other distortions. These alternative research designs are called "observational studies." For example, cohort studies follow a group of subjects over time, relying on statistical modeling to seek associations with the development of particular outcomes. Case-control studies probe attributes of cases that might be lacking in people who are spared the particular health effect. A cross-sectional study takes a snapshot of a population at a given time and tries to discern if those who have the health effect at issue differ from those who don't.

All these designs are far simpler and less costly than RCTs because they accept the subjects as they find them, but all have serious inherent shortcomings. Some of the shortcomings can be overcome by meticulous attention to the details of the study and analysis, but no amount of fiddle can overcome their inherent weaknesses. They are quick, down-and-dirty ways to test a clinical hypothesis. If they are done as well as possible and the result is inconclusive, it's time to move on to another hypothesis. If they are promising and you care, it's time to move on to an RCT. I am certainly not alone in my qualms about observational studies. However, no observational study can demonstrate efficacy; that requires an RCT. And without reassurance that an intervention works in some group of patients, there is no logical way to know whether interventions monitored in observational studies are better than nothing, or even worse than nothing. Hence, we are going to focus on evidence for efficacy from RCTs in all our policy considerations.

Notions of efficacy and effectiveness are crucial to the design of a rational health-care system. They are also readily subverted by the purposes of marketing, and not just direct-to-consumer marketing. The hawking of pharmaceutical wares always claims significant benefit. The consumer has to ask: benefit for what, and how much benefit? The claim of significant benefit is nearly always based on a statistically significant difference, which is nearly always illustrated with an effect expressed in relative terms, for example, a 50 percent decrease in some evil outcome. If the efficacy was such that half of all people treated are benefited, one is duly impressed. If the intervention reduced the incidence of the health effect from 8 in 1,000 to 4 in 1,000—also a 50 percent decrease—are you impressed? That's why the notion of the number need to treat (NNT) to help one patient has taken hold; it is much more intuitively obvious, as is the number needed to treat to harm one patient (NNH).

To make an informed medical decision, one needs more than the NNH and NNT. One needs to know how much one is likely to be benefited or harmed. You might have an agent that produces an effect in most, but that's less compelling if the effect is trivial. It also matters a great deal if the benefit is a surrogate outcome (such as a risk factor) or the clinical process itself. Many drugs are licensed because statistically significant but clinically trivial effects have been massaged out of trial data. I call this "small effectology." Most of these drugs are hawked with language that is designed to fool the listener. All this needs to be appreciated for the sophistry it represents.

Statistical evidence for efficacy, not the degree of efficacy and not effectiveness, is the primary consideration in the studies of the Cochrane Collaboration, and it is the critical factor in licensing decisions for pharmaceuticals at the FDA. Thus evidence for any efficacy is the hypothesis tested in nearly all industry-sponsored RCTs. Of all the organizations and agencies in the world of evidence-based medicine, only the American College of Physician's ACP Journal Club has been emphasizing whether the evidence of efficacy is meaningful in terms of NNTs. Recently, the U.S. Preventive Services Task Force has moved in this direction. There is a utilitarian rationale for accepting evidence for small degrees of efficacy as persuasive, even determinative, because it can translate into considerable effectiveness—in theory. The efficacy may seem minimal, even trivial, from the perspective of a given individual but may be sizable for the population at large. Hence, an NNT of 250 may spare a sizable number of people if millions are treated. Generalizing from an RCT to the burden of disease in the population follows from the pioneering work of epidemiologist Geoffrey Rose (*The Strategy of Preventive Medicine* [1992]) but takes liberties I am not prepared to accept. It assumes that RCTs can be powered (in a statistical sense) to discern small effects reliably. As I detail in chapter 3, unavoidable and immeasurable error in the way subjects are randomized and much more should make everyone as wary as it makes me dismissive.

If we were to power trials for large degrees of efficacy based on some a priori consensus as to what is valuable, the size, duration, and cost of RCTs would decrease dramatically, and their reproducibility would increase. Several such high-efficacy trials could probe for efficacy in subsets of patients: young, old, with confounders and without. We'd no longer be studying tens of thousands of subjects for years in the hopes of being able to dredge evidence for some small effect out of the morass of data. Rather, efficacy of a high degree (a large effect) would translate into effectiveness for the subset studied.

The argument against efficient RCTs seeking such evidence for efficacy relates to adverse effects. RCTs for high degrees of efficacy offer an assessment of short-term, highly frequent adverse effects. However, such RCTs are unlikely to detect adverse effects that might be only moderately less frequent than the health effect being sought, or that are frequent in subjects that might not have qualified for the RCT because they didn't quite meet the criteria for entry (maybe they were too old or too young, had another disease, etc.). This is the "first, do no harm" argument, and it's a telling argument. However, the only way to monitor for lesser and less-frequent events in a spectrum of exposed patients is with efficient post-marketing surveillance. This was one of many recommendations in the 2007 Institute of Medicine proposal for reforming the FDA and its regulatory role, to which the FDA has responded in part. The proposal for reform that I am leading up to in this chapter offers a much more global approach to pharmacosurveillance.

Devices, Procedures, and the Risk/Benefit Ratio

The next institution that we must confront is the industry supporting the design and manufacture of new medical devices, the topic of chapter 4. The Supreme Court decision in *Riegel v. Medtronic* protects manufacturers from torts for harm caused by devices that have negotiated the gentle barrier to licensure by the FDA. This removes the plaintiff's bar from the safety equation. No doubt, there will still be suits relating to manufacturing flaws and operator errors, but the Supreme Court is assuming that licensure of a device by the FDA is prima facie reassurance of safety; reassurance of efficacy is a secondary consideration, one that the FDA assigns in large part to operator judgment and competence. Looking on the bright side, perhaps little is lost since the plaintiff's bar was a very inefficient remedy. It is inefficient procedurally, since closure in one venue may mean little for another. Product-liability litigation is a difficult pill for the courts when medical devices are at issue; the distinction between an adverse outcome and an adverse effect is seldom unequivocal in a given patient.

It is time for the FDA and the public in general to demand as much rigor in licensing indwelling devices for elective procedures as for pharmaceuticals. That means that scientific evidence for efficacy is a requisite for licensure. If there is a standard, tried-and-true device, there should be head-to-head RCTs demonstrating a meaningful reason to switch to the newer device and mandatory surveillance for adverse events once it is licensed. An example of this is the hardware for total hip replacements. Many a surgeon has devised a new component and retained patent rights and royalties in the process. We are now seeing the disaster of the "metal on metal" hip, which was implanted in many unsuspecting patients, only to learn that the device is far less durable than promised and that the tried-and-true older versions were better. We should never license an indwelling device if the result of the RCT is less than a meaningful improvement over the standard treatment; a result suggesting equivalence or "noninferiority" in the short term does not justify the uncertainties about problems in the future. Innovation for innovation's sake is not good.

I also am very wary of head-to-head trials. If there is a device (or a pharmaceutical) that is clearly effective, then it becomes the gold standard for treatment. RCTs would be designed to compare a novel approach with this gold standard. It would be unethical to compare the novel device with a placebo and thereby deprive the control group of a treatment known to treat their condition effectively. The choice to study the novel treatment head-to-head is as ethically demanding as the choice to give patients a placebo. Two questions must be answered before initiating a head-to-head trial. First, how golden is the gold standard? If the gold standard itself is barely effective, a demonstration that the novel intervention is equivalent is worth little. And second, if the gold standard is effective, how much more effective must the novel intervention be to justify exposing patients to unknown long-term risks?

The history of the introduction of surgical interventions for low back pain is an object lesson. Since almost no intervention has proved efficacious, let alone effective, there is no gold standard. There are standards of care that rely on consensus rather than science. And there are numerous examples of head-to-head trials comparing an investigator's technological brainstorm with the investigator's notion of standard of care. All the novel forms of disc removal, spine fusion, and disc replacement have been compared with the usual surgical procedure in head-to-head trials, yielding equivocal results in terms of efficacy. Always the investigator declares the result a success because the procedure is no worse than the standard of care but stands on more sound theoretical footings—that is, the investigator's preconceptions. The few trials, mainly from Europe, that compare the surgical intervention with conservative treatment are consistent with the interpretation that all one is afforded by spine surgery is an NNH, not an NNT.

Any suggestion that a placebo-controlled surgical trial is necessary to establish efficacy is anathema on ethical grounds if the outcome is life or death. In such cases, the standard of care is the best one can do, and advances must be layered cautiously on top of the standard. But many interventions, such as those for back pain and coronary artery disease, are not sparing one from imminent death or damage. These interventions are designed to provide relief of symptoms: less pain and improved function in the short term with hope for more-substantive advantages in the longer term. Furthermore, invasive interventions for symptom relief are even more prone to placebo effects (chapter 6) than are pharmaceuticals or physical treatments. An RCT that compares an invasive procedure with a less-invasive placebo introduces considerable bias toward the putative efficacy of the procedure. The only control that obviates this bias would be a sham procedure.

I have no ethical reservations regarding sham-controlled trials. These are interventions designed to improve symptoms, not overt damage such as escalating kidney disease or the like, which can be objectively quantified. If there is no efficacious gold standard for head-to-head comparison, if the risks of the sham procedure are minimized, if consent is truly informed, and if the risks are justified by the potential value of the science, sham-controlled RCTs are ethical. In fact, given the tragedy that is modern spine surgery and modern invasive cardiology, licensing indwelling devices and condoning invasive procedures without scientific testing is unethical.

The standard for the licensure of indwelling devices or elective surgical procedures should be as stringent as for novel pharmaceuticals. We, the professionals, need to come to grips with the reason for stringency. Citizen Patients should demand that we do.

Patient-Oriented Clinimetrics and the Contract Research Organization

The last institution we will confront in this section is relatively new: the Contract Research Organization (CRO). A new drug application (NDA) to the FDA is a hefty document. At its core is the analysis of at least one RCT, which purports statistically significant evidence that the drug is as good as, if not better than, a placebo or any alternative drug. The licensing process involves convincing the FDA that this assertion of evidence is tenable and the need for the agent compelling. For most NDAs today, the manufacturer has outsourced much of the application, including the RCT itself. The application process has spawned a multibillion-dollar industry of companies that contract to perform the RCT, analyze the data, and assist the pharmaceutical firm in preparing and defending the NDA.

There are many of these CROs, some of which are integrated into academic health centers (see chapter 1). I have had, and have voiced, concerns about this arrangement from the start, and I was there at the start. The patriarch of the CRO industry was junior faculty with me, a colleague who collaborated on research projects and a book before his consulting to the pharmaceutical industry grew into Quintiles Transnational, Inc. My qualms about the marriage between pharmaceutical firms and CROs relate to conflicts of interest. So much has been written about this issue that I need not further decry the fashion in which the pharmaceutical industry's business model is driven by profits and profit margins. The CRO functions in the service of that business model.

Science tests null hypotheses: a negative result is assumed and a positive result is a surprise. The pharmaceutical industry's business model wants and expects a positive result and is disappointed when none is forthcoming. This is often a very costly disappointment; one might well imagine, then, that a positive result would be more conducive than a negative result to the manufacturer negotiating another contract with the CRO. A negative result might make a competing CRO seem more appealing. Nearly all modern RCTs are designed to demonstrate a small, albeit statistically significant, degree of efficacy. Given the judgment involved in analyzing the enormous data sets generated by these large RCTs, one need not postulate malfeasance to imagine some prejudice at work. There is no mystery that whenever one compares RCTs supported by industry with RCTs supported by public moneys for the same drug, the same class of drug, and even for meta-analyses on the same class of drug, the industry-supported studies are more likely to be positive.

We are institutionalizing conflicts of interest. It starts with the fashion in which RCTs are outsourced, percolates down to the academic health centers, and passes on through the "thought leaders" to the practicing doctors. We can do much if we tackle the fountainhead. We will go a long way just by demanding that efficacy trials seek only clinically important health effects. It's much harder to torture data to produce a large effect than to produce a small effect, and I don't value the latter. It is time to call a halt to "small effectology."

I am ambivalent about the advocacy for continuing an exclusively private-sector pharmaceutical industry. It is argued that profit is a motivator for innovation and for efficiency. The argument rests on historical precedent, such as the Nobel Prize–winning discovery of therapeutic antimetabolites by George Hitchings and Gertrude Elion while working at Burroughs-Wellcome pharmaceutical company. However, very few such basic innovations have spilled out of the research laboratories of the pharmaceutical industry in the past couple of decades. Most of the critical and novel advances in basic science have been the brainchildren of scientists working in federal laboratories (such as the NIH in the United States and MRC Laboratories in the United Kingdom) or in the academy, usually with federal funding. The contributions of scientists employed in the pharmaceutical industry have been more in the realm of finding applications for these advances rather than generating the insights in the first place. It is in this activity that competition and market share are motivators that drive efficiency. Sadly, we have learned that efficacy can be no match for market share. One way to rein in this dialectic is to designate the licensing of such products as a public-sector function and delegate the responsibility to the FDA and similar agencies in other countries.

Protecting Considerations of Efficacy from Conflicts of Interest

As detailed in earlier chapters, the flaws in this algorithm have become all too obvious. Because of this track record, I argue that modern RCTs should also be a public-sector responsibility. I suggest the establishment of clinimetrics centers at medical schools and national RCT steering committees. All these entities should be staffed by academicians committed to the relevant issues in epidemiology. There is no shortage of willing and competent academics in schools of public health, as well as in the clinical faculties. Funding for the staffing should be from federal coffers; the cost will be more than compensated by the savings that derive from keeping ineffective and me-too drugs from the nation's medicine chests. The steering committees would prioritize RCTs by therapeutic promise and need and offer the clinimetrics centers the opportunity to bid to participate. The clinimetrics centers would function as public CROs and as the only agent to prepare and submit the NDAs. In our youth, before he founded Quintiles, Dennis Gillings and I formulated a very efficient RCT design that called for treating a small number of centers, each with a small number of subjects, as individual data points ("On the Design of the Phase III Drug Trial," *Arthritis and Rheumatism* 26 [1983]: 1354–61).

Such a design speaks to the generalizability of results while rendering the process of testing for efficacy so much more efficient than what is going on today. It also passes the principal cost of drug development on to the taxpayer up front. The present system is an excuse for the overinflated pricing of pharmaceuticals, the cost of which is assumed by taxpayers in the cost of Medicare.

The Insurance Industry and the Many Moral Hazards

The insurance industry is its own fortress, but we must confront it. In the conventional wisdom, health-insurance companies have our interests at heart and at the forefront of their business models. That was my assumption, too, but no vestige of naïveté remains today. The needs, wants, and expectations of the clients, claimants, and beneficiaries are barely discernible and certainly not high priority in today's corporate models and corporate ethics. The majority of the people in the United States who have health or workers' compensation insurance are insured by their employer and serviced by their insurance company. A minority are self-insured individuals who are serviced by their insurance company. I am in the majority that is insured by their employer. So if I need heart transplantation, Blue Cross Blue Shield of North Carolina passes that $500,000 cost on to my employer, the state of North Carolina, as an addition to the premium. The insurance company negotiates a fee for processing claims (some percentage of the total cost) and takes that off the top of the money that flows from the employer through the insurance-company coffers to the providers. If I were self-employed and purchased my own policy, the pool of the self-insured would be expected to cover the additional expense of the heart transplant. That's why my policy costs the state some $6,000 per year, whereas it would cost three to four times that amount if I were to purchase it on my own. But that's the least of the unsavory features.

The former arrangement, in which the employer is essentially self-insured, creates a conflict for the insurer. The more money spent on "health care" by the insured, the more money (in processing fees) flows into the coffers of the insurer, which pays the enormous salaries and other aspects of "overhead" that are features of this industry whether the entity is legally profit making or nominally "not-for-profit." Why do you think the health-insurance companies are so willing to promote screening programs and to underwrite the most expensive of me-too agents and unproved devices and procedures? Nearly all screening, from cholesterol to PSA to mammography, leads to marginal benefit, if any, for the screened but generates much largesse for the screeners and even more for the underwriters.

The Centers for Medicare and Medicaid Services (CMS), which administers Medicare, is faced with enormous political pressures as to what should be covered and at what cost. A single-payer insurance system is long overdue, but even in such a system, the issue would be who decides what is to be paid for and how much should be paid. Imagine the escalation in the activities of lobbyists and political action committees (PACs) if the single payer were to be a federal agency. The response to the U.S. Preventive Services Task Force recommendations on mammography and PSA screening was swift and loud. And that was just in response to a recommendation. If the CMS were to attempt to structure coverage based on efficacy, heads would roll. That's why the CMS backed away from refusing to pay for vertebroplasty following the two negative sham-controlled RCTs (chapter 6). That's why all the tinkering with Medicare involves administrative change rather than tackling the substance of coverage.

Then there's the most egregious of the insurance models: the model for workers' compensation. Again, the majority of the expense is taken on by the large employers who insure the larger workforces. Again, the insurance company profits when more claims are processed. However, this industry has an actuarial model for disability insurance. The business model demands that all funds be collected at the outset to cover the pension for the duration of any long-term disability. These firms have war chests that we tend to learn about only in economic downturns when their investments sour. As long as industry can pay the premiums, there is no financial disincentive for workers' compensation insurers to truly reform the accountability of the provision of care and of disability determination. This is an indemnity scheme that commandeers 3 to 8 percent of wages and consumes some 80 percent of this largesse at the expense of the health and prognosis of claimants who find their backache or arm pain disabling. They are cash cows for the workers' compensation insurance industry, which returns the favor in the form of long-term invalidity.

The rationale for insurance is that we share the risks of the catastrophes that might befall and decimate any one of us. In the early days of the insurance industry, there were fears that someone who needed money would torch his or her house, the so-called "moral-hazard" argument. The moral-hazard concept pertained to the claimant. That's not how I see it today. The moral hazard pertains much more to the other stakeholders to varying degrees. We all share the cost of overtreatment and guilt for allowing its persistence. No one pays the price more than the worker who suffers from regional musculoskeletal disorders, a price that is measured in unnecessary and ill-advised interventions that result in prolonged suffering.

Finally, a word about tort insurance. A tort is a lawsuit brought to right a wrong. It works well for many a wrong, but not so well for a personal injury in which "pain and suffering" constitutes the consequence of the wrong. Much is known of the illness experience itself, and much is known about the personal price one pays for redress for this aspect of a personal injury; but it is clear that these two are simply incompatible. The illness experience calls for coping skills; seeking redress encourages one to magnify symptoms. Alleviation of symptoms in the former is a triumph; in the latter, it is costly. As a result, redress for "pain and suffering" is as elusive as escalation of "pain and suffering" is predictable. No-fault schemes are a better way.

Assuring Health, Insuring Disease

I have been honing an approach to rational reform of the health-care system based on the above considerations for some time. The effort takes advantage of insights gained from firsthand analysis of the sociopolitical constraints placed on clinical judgment in many countries. It takes into account the analysis of medicalization and Type II Medical Malpractice I have put forth in earlier books, and it takes into account all that has been put forth in this book.

Most models for reform are not viable because of fiscal and political constraints. I have presented earlier versions to a number of leading scholars and several state agencies. And I have published earlier iterations that were designed to be a private-sector alternative and to be offered to the uninsured workforce. I have neither heard, nor can I conjure up, a substantive criticism to this approach, but I was not surprised when pressures were brought to squelch it, even in the lone state in which legislation tolerates innovation for the uninsured workforce. I am fully aware that this is not a fine-tuning or tweaking but a thoroughgoing change that would dramatically affect the incomes and lifestyles of almost everyone gainfully involved in the status quo. Very few would come out better financially. However, all would find their roles clarified and their souls cleansed by putting the health and welfare of the citizenry first. All would earn gratitude and respect by participating in a service profession that truly serves others. The pride in and pleasure from working in health care has eroded in the past fifty years. It will return. I may not live long enough to see it through to fulfillment, but I can hope to see it stir.

Given the experience with private-sector reform, I propose a state-based system for assuring health and insuring disease. The less-populous states may need to cooperate to reach a critical mass of more than 10 million people, but it is important that the national system operate as a conglomerate of independent units. This has nothing to do with market considerations; I have no need to demonstrate yet again that free-market principles do not apply to health care in the United States. Rather, the multiplication in the system is to serve the range of philosophies of well-being that this reform countenances.

Each state would create a fund, an Enablement Fund. It may be more palatable, given the precedents, if this fund were a percentage of wages—12 percent—but a comparable fund could derive from income taxation. By comparison, this is far less than we currently expend on "health insurance." The moneys would distribute to two accounts, a Disease Insurance Account and a Health Assurance Account. The Disease Insurance Account is a shared-risk pool designed to supplant health insurance as we know it until one is eligible for federal Medicare insurance. The Health Assurance Account is not a shared risk pool. It is the repository for all moneys not expended from the Disease Insurance Account. Ownership in the Health Assurance Account would be prorated to contributions. That account would be available for licensed services in the state relating to health that are not underwritten by the Disease Insurance Account. This will become clear below.

DISEASE INSURANCE ACCOUNT

The intellectual engine for managing the Disease Insurance Account would be the same local clinimetrics center discussed above as participating in multisite RCTs testing new interventions for clinically meaningful efficacy. The professional staff of the clinimetrics center would include dedicated full-time epidemiologists and statisticians, along with rotating full-time clinicians with epidemiology training and bent. As mentioned before, there is no manpower shortage. There would be regulations that declare the accepting of gifts, consultative fees, and the like by the staff to be illegal activities. The process must be as free of conflicts of interest as possible. There would be two safeguards built into the system. One relates to the ability to compare administrative decisions across the states. The other follows from the clinimetrics center's fiduciary role. The size of the

Enablement Fund would be fixed by the gross domestic product (GDP) of the state. The administration of the Disease Insurance Account could not spend more than the fund has available. Furthermore, the administration could not "save" money; money not expended in the Disease Insurance Account would revert to the Health Assurance Account.

The guiding principle of the Disease Insurance Account is to indemnify all that is demonstrated to have clinically meaningful efficacy. The exercise is to calculate NNTs by taking advantage of evidence statements from the Cochrane Collaboration, the ACP Journal Club, the FDA's trial-data repository, and whatever else might be relevant without duplicating these available and ongoing evidence exercises. Agreeing on prerequisite NNTs for effectiveness requires a good deal of consensus building in each clinimetrics center.

1. There is variability in the magnitude of effect between the trials that find evidence for efficacy. Hence, there is often a range of NNTs.

2. What NNT does one need in order to declare the efficacy clinically meaningful? I, and most others who are students of this exercise, would argue that an NNT of 50 is the upper limit of reliability and of meaningfulness for an unequivocal, easy-to-quantify outcome such as death, heart attack, etc. This means that a physician would need to treat 50 people for 1 to stand a good chance of benefiting. I would personally be more comfortable with an NNT of 20 or less for my cutoff. This is an issue in philosophy (and cost, as we'll discuss), but it is also an issue in the effect being measured. These cutoffs are defensible when the outcome is "hard"—that is, unequivocal, such as death, heart attack, end-stage renal disease, and the like. But here, too, there is a proviso. The effect has to be clinically meaningful in the context of life-course epidemiology. If the intervention spares 1 person in 20 from death by colon cancer but spares none of these from death from something else at the same time (all-cause mortality), the clinically meaningful NNT is not 20 since there is no meaningful result. Death is death.

3. NNTs for "soft" outcomes are more problematic. How much better do you have to make patients with rheumatoid arthritis feel, and how many patients have to feel better, before you would consider the efficacy to be clinically meaningful? That depends in part on the reliability and validity of the measure of subjective improvement. If there is a reasonable measure, how many more patients must improve when treated with an active agent rather than

with a placebo or an old standby? Again, before analytic modeling is sensible, consensus must be reached as to the quality of these measures and their relevance to clinical efficacy. That consensus will always be more severe than for "hard" outcomes; NNTs of 5 resonate with me. That means an end to "me-too" drugs.

4. The derivation and analysis of NNTs must be undertaken for a large but finite number of interventions and then must be repeated periodically as new data appear. I suspect a well-staffed clinimetrics center could handle a quarter of the clinical circumstances each year. Realize that most analyses find evidence lacking or absent, thereby rendering the efficacy exercise perfunctory.

The clinimetrics center would have two other functions relating to the Disease Insurance Account. First, a good deal of the practice of medicine that is "common practice" has never been subjected to scientific testing and may never be. Is such to be indemnified, and to what extent? Second, the center has to interact with the national RCT steering committee regarding participation in RCTs to test the efficacy of new agents and devices.

A prime example of common practice is the clinical interview. The clinical interview is the essence of the medical treatment act. Furthermore, as I will make clear in the next chapter, the clinical interview is the basis for a therapeutic relationship. The physician has to listen to the "chief complaint," place that complaint into a clinical context, and act on the context. Some of the process can be subjected to scientific testing as to efficacy, efficiency, reliability, and even effectiveness. But not all can be studied. The clinical interview does much more than collect data relevant to the differential diagnosis; it establishes the trust that is necessary for medical decision making. True, medical decision making is simplified by expunging the ineffective from the menu that is indemnified.

Some might argue that computerized decision aids are the answer, but I am a serious doubter, and I am in good company. I suspect that "decision aids" will be useful only when the decision lends itself to the kind of analytic approach the clinimetrics center is taking to the issue of efficacy. The clinimetrics center is a de facto decision aid. There is much more to the experience of illness, however, from semiotics to the making of decisions when the data are inadequate. That is when you need a physician. I would argue that everyone should have an hour of medical interview underwritten for each year of adult life. If you don't need a clinical interview until you're forty, you will have accumulated nineteen (or more, depending on the definition of adulthood) hours of clinical interview time to be used as needed. I mean "as needed," since, based on NNTs, there is no reason to underwrite a routine annual examination. If one is worried, though, that is a legitimate "need" and one that may be well served.

Another prime example of common practice that is not as common as it should be is psychological counseling. The American saga of regional low back pain would not be as convoluted if some or all could find their way into productive counseling. There are RCTs of forms of talk therapy, cognitive behavior therapy in particular, for a number of psychological challenges from insomnia to fatigue that demonstrate a degree of efficacy. No one has been able to design a trial that demonstrates compelling efficacy of such counseling, let alone cost-effectiveness, because of all the vagaries related to practice style, client differences, and outcome measures. As with the clinical interview, though, I am strongly prejudiced toward a belief in the value of "talk therapy" with someone who is prepared to be helpful. It is not expensive. For the salary of one overpaid hospital administrator, you could hire ten to twenty social workers, give each a caseload of ten to twenty struggling families, and, even if only a minority were helped, make a very important difference. And for one year of useless interventional cardiology and cardiovascular surgery at my hospital, we could employ great teams of social workers. Therefore, in my plan, everyone insured under the Disease Insurance Account would be underwritten for a cumulative annual evaluative hour and short-term intervention when indicated.

The clinimetrics centers will be offered the opportunity to participate in RCTs that have been prioritized by the national RCT steering committees and designed to test whether a new intervention fails to produce clinically meaningful efficacy. Agreeing to be a participating center is a challenging and complex decision. The center will be recruiting patients from its catchment area, organizing data collection and analysis, and paying for patient care. The last is less of a burden for a pharmaceutical since the agent is supplied gratis from the manufacturer, but monitoring for adverse and salutary effects can be expensive. For RCTs of devices and procedures, the underwriting can entail substantial sums for patient care. "Finder fees" and other inducements will be history once the ethics of this approach to medical progress is incorporated into the fabric of American life. So the clinimetrics center has to revisit the thinking of the national RCT steering committee. If the agent under study proves clinically efficacious, will it be of enough value to enough people in the state account to justify participating in the trial, or are resources better spent participating in a different trial?

Speaking of money and resources, there is no doubt that there will be enormous savings when the Enablement Fund replaces the current mess. The bizarrely expensive business of NDAs will be streamlined. The marketing and "educational" budgets of manufacturers and providers will become transparent and easy to regulate. Many of the currently available elective high-ticket items will no longer be underwritten. They will be cut off by their ephemeral NNTs, not by their pricing or anything else that smacks of rationing. Based on the analysis of the topics considered in my earlier books, the per capita annual expenditure from the Disease Insurance Account today would not exceed half of the moneys in the Enablement Fund with the current pricing schedule. Furthermore, starting this account from scratch allows for innovative and cost-saving Internet technologies that will eliminate a good deal of the current administrative overhead.

The Disease Insurance Account also is in a position to be very proactive in regard to cost-effectiveness beyond excluding the ineffective. There is no reason to tolerate the repugnant incomes garnered by the many administrators currently employed in the American "health-care" industry. The Disease Insurance Account can stipulate the overhead percentage it is willing to underwrite. Furthermore, it is straightforward to add cost to the NNT by applying the COPE (cost of preventing an event) statistic, which factors the cost of the treatment into the NNT. There is no reason why the account could not negotiate with purveyors based on the cost-effectiveness of the intervention. For example, TNF-alpha inhibitors are biotechnology triumphs that lead to important symptomatic improvement in about half of patients with active rheumatoid arthritis unresponsive to traditional agents. These are efficacious agents. They cost well over $10,000 per year. Rheumatoid arthritis afflicts 1 percent of the population but is not a severe progressive disease in most. The agents are marvels, but the intellectual wherewithal to develop them derived from Nobel and Lasker Award–winning contributions from government-supported laboratories. There is no advantage to the Disease Insurance Account to underwrite the marketing budgets of the manufacturers, or their "educational budgets," or the outrageousness of their profit margin. An NNT-COPE calculation would justify a price that is a fraction of the current price, and the Disease Insurance Account should demand such in a very public fashion.

Notice I am not recommending the stipulation of "co-pay." If the intervention is efficacious, it's provided. However, I fear as great a backlash from stakeholders in the current system, including all the providers and purveyors of the ineffective—a backlash that could prove litigious. My solution is to have two levels of co-pay: 0 or 100 percent. If the patient insists on something that is not covered and therefore requires 100 percent co-pay because it is deemed to offer inadequate effectiveness, he or she will be so informed, and informed as well that there is a fallback in the Health Assurance Account, as we'll discuss. Notice, too, that I am not countenancing stratified health care. The Disease Insurance Account underwrites what is efficacious for patients whether employed, unemployed, injured, or disabled. Any intervention proven to offer sufficient efficacy that had been indemnified by Medicaid, workers' compensation, and private "health" insurance will now be indemnified by the Disease Insurance Account. Ethical medical ministration knows no such distinctions.

HEALTH ASSURANCE ACCOUNT

As I have noted, health is difficult to define. I take comfort in the fact that even the late Hans-Georg Gadamer, a twentieth-century philosopher of great reputation, said: "The fundamental fact remains that it is illness and not health which 'objectifies' itself, which confronts us as something opposed to us and which forces itself on us. . . . The real mystery lies in the hidden character of health." Health is still an enigma, but not the enigma it once was. Life-course epidemiology has unraveled some of the mystery, though not the underlying mechanisms. Health in the resource-advantaged world requires the wherewithal to feel comfortable in your skin. You need to find a station in your community that satisfies to an important degree. You need to be able to maintain that station by virtue of the earnings from work that satisfies to an important degree. You need to have the personal resources to cope with the predicaments that are bound to come up. High on this list of predicaments are the occasional encounter with painful episodes, and regional low back pain is firmly and prominently entrenched among these, along with heartache, headache, and heartburn. Health does not require low cholesterol, low blood pressure, low body mass index, normal kidney function, normal cardiac output, etc. It is the erosion of these that is prerequisite to disease. You can have rheumatoid arthritis and still have your health if you are a *person* with rheumatoid arthritis and not a "rheumatoid."

The Health Assurance Account exists to foster health. It accumulates based on an individual's contribution to the Enablement Fund minus the expenditures of the Disease Insurance Account. It is managed like a state retirement fund so that it accrues in value similarly to other managed funds. But it is yours on a prorated basis to do whatever you wish related to health (as defined above) that is provided by licensed professionals in your state. If you never touch it, it will revert to your pension at retirement. If you are not convinced that cholesterol screening or coronary artery stents are as ineffective as determined by the clinimetrics center, you can use your Health Assurance Account funds toward the purchase of such outside the Disease Insurance Account. And if you want to purchase a treatment act or modality that is not covered by the Disease Insurance Account because it is no more effective than a placebo or because it is designed to "work" as a placebo, you can feel free to do so. These are your moneys. No one else is sharing the cost.

The Health Assurance Account will have an advisory component. If you are an entry-level employee, it might be very wise for you to expend Health Assurance funds for instruction in English as a second language or to acquire skills that afford job mobility. These moneys are available to aid you if you don't otherwise have the wherewithal for attaining a station in life that promotes your healthfulness. There is a role for the Disease Insurance Account in educating the public as to the hazards of not attaining a satisfying station in life, thereby making it more sensible and, hopefully, less necessary to expend Health Assurance funds for this purpose.

The Future of Fee-for-Service

"Fee-for-service" is a modern, and largely American, notion that arose during the past century. In the Middle Ages in Europe, physicians had a "public calling" and received a voluntary "honorarium" for ministering to the ill and dying. The principle of a "public calling" was inculcated in the Prussian social legislation that was the template for national health-insurance schemes across the industrial world—except in the United States. As I mentioned earlier in the chapter, national health insurance almost made landfall here in the platform of the Progressive (Bull Moose) Party but was squelched with the defeat of Theodore Roosevelt in the presidential election of 1912. The AMA supported the Progressive Platform but, shortly after its defeat, did an about-face. In 1923 the AMA Code of Medical Ethics allowed that the physician is "free to choose whom he will serve." And the code in 1957 allowed that physician fees should be "commensurate with the services rendered and the patient's ability to pay." This was the era of "sliding scales" and "soak the rich." It was the era of charity wards and of the frail and not-so-elderly dying destitute at home. It was an era that came to the end with the enactment of Medicare. In 1980 the AMA Code of Medical Ethics contains no allusion to a sliding scale.

Chapter 2 details the politics of this transition. Neither the AMA nor its constituents would yield on the principle of "fee-for-service" or relinquish the physician's prerogative regarding what is necessary and appropriate care. Hence, President Johnson struck a Faustian deal in order to spare Americans from a mean old age. The Medicare legislation called for committees of physicians and surgeons to define all of the above, including "customary" and "reasonable" charges. Chapter 2 explains the workings of the Current Procedural Terminology (CPT) Editorial Panel and the Resource-based Relative Value Scale Update Committee (RUC). However, this institutionalization of self-service is running into the harsh realities of fiscal constraint. Every medical specialty and subspecialty organization and their fellow travelers are lobbying Congress furiously to preserve their particular turf. It's inelegant behavior, if not downright ugly.

Of all their arguments, the weakest is to preserve fee-for-service. That's because of the evolution of the notion of "service" that I described in chapter 2. It is most readily quantified in terms of things done to patients, particularly procedures. If that's all there is to "service," then market forces have a ready foothold. For example, there are two excellent randomized trials comparing colonoscopy performed by gastroenterologists with that performed by nurse practitioners. Their performance is indistinguishable. Furthermore, their competence, or lack thereof, should they create a catastrophe (such as perforate the colon) is indistinguishable; both would have to yell for a surgeon. The dramatic difference is that the nurse practitioners performed as part of their salaried duties; the gastroenterologists charge more than $2,000 for this "service." Since many procedures are performed by video monitoring, perhaps the skills of the young soldiers in Houston who fly drones in South Asia can be harnessed for all sorts of procedures at a distance, with technicians following their instructions.

Fee-for-service is difficult to defend in the twenty-first century. I'd rather see an attempt to defend "fee-for-serving" or "fee-for-professionalism." Isn't an orthopedist as valuable for informing a patient that she will not be advantaged by screwing her spine up as for doing the screwing? If we have the debate on the value of "serving" and the value of "professionalism," we might see the role of the physician in modern society in a positive light. If not, we may not see a role for a physician at all.

It's a very long tunnel, but there is a positive light at the end. And that light is shining on a "clinic" we can be proud of once again.

A Clinic for the
Twenty-First Century

I am a student of the history of Western medicine and of its practice. That history is not without serious failings and failures, but it is also a history of an ideal, of intelligent people earning the mantle of "physician" and devoting their lives to bringing compassion, the wisdom of their time, and the science of their day to the aid of those who are ill. I have aspired to such a role for as long as I can remember, and I have worked toward this goal ever since I became a physician in 1968. I know no higher calling, and I have found it impossible to stand by and watch the erosion of this calling in my lifetime.

The Citizen Patient is the fifth book I have written about the discordance between the evidentiary basis for medical practice and the reality of medical practice in America. My goal with the first four is to inform medical decision making. But the passion that serves as the engine for this book is to champion the ideals of my profession and its professionalism for the benefit of generations to come. *The Citizen Patient* details the sociopolitical constraints that have come to pummel these ideals and offers an example of a programmatic remedy. We stand at a time in the history of the profession of medicine when its highest calling might finally be fulfilled. This chapter is written to describe what would result if we cast off out-of-date notions and misguided practices and move the care of the patient into a clinic appropriate for the twenty-first century.

What the "Doc-in-the-Box" and the "In-Store Clinic" Won't Do for You

I suppose there are medical conditions that can be diagnosed and treated in the abstract, without even seeing you, let alone talking to you or laying hands on you. If you accept the pronouncements of august organizations, you might submit to a screening examination or vaccination with the provider knowing nothing more than your name and insurance status. Or if you suffer damage from physical trauma, why not just get it fixed? Or if you have an obvious infection, why not take an antibiotic? Does it matter who you are? In such circumstances, isn't any impedance to fixing or treating simply meddlesome, something that leads to greater expense and loss of time? This is the principle that fuels the exploding doc-in-the-box movement.

Clinics are budding in retail stores or their parking lots across the land, usually staffed by allied health professionals with physician "oversight." These are designed as volume providers of the obvious. They are Patients-R-Us. And they are a very shortsighted and narrow-minded approach to the challenge of providing an alternative to the cumbersome and expensive American system.

The underlying premise that illness can ever be objectified is flawed. Take the example of "minor" trauma. Sure, this is likely the result of an accident. But that assumption will miss abusive relationships or predisposing musculoskeletal or neurologic impairments. Seldom is the treatment of "minor infections" simply reflexive. There are important reasons to consider options for ear, "sinus," urinary tract, and skin infections. And many vaccination and screening programs are much more controversial than one is led to believe.

For me, a visit to the clinic is not an exercise in cookbook medicine or in treating common things because they are common. The clinic has a higher calling. "Clinic" does not denote a physical space, a building, or a room with benches. "Clinic" is the meeting of the minds of one patient and one physician. Physicians don't simply go to "clinic"; they have "clinic" and hold "clinic," and they have long done so.

Traditionally, the clinic was a hallowed ground, a priestly purview in which the patient felt like a supplicant. "The clinic," asserts Michel Foucault in *The Birth of the Clinic* (1963), "was this constant gaze upon the patient, this age-old, yet ever renewed attention that enabled medicine not to disappear entirely with each new speculation, but to preserve itself, to assume little by little the figure of a truth that is definitive, if not completed, in short, to develop below the level of the noisy episodes of its history, in a continuous historicity. In the non-variable of the clinic, medicine . . . bound truth and time together." Every person who entered such a psychological space felt a degree of trepidation. Even a physician who entered this space as a patient found their priestly aura stripped away. No one left such a space without being wilted by the experience.

But this need not and should not be so any longer. Medicine in the twenty-first century can serve brilliantly without relying on rituals, auras, and paternalism. Doctor and patient can be collaborators. Licensure and other credentialing should assure competence, not exclusivity.

Don't think for one moment that converting the clinic from sermon to colloquy is a foregone conclusion, however. Discarding the robes of medical priesthood is to discard an advantage that has been self-preserving and self-aggrandizing for generations. And for medicine to discard the vestiges of the guild system is to assume vulnerability in terms of authority—and of income. If this new "clinic" is to come to pass, it is because the modern patient understands why it should and exercises the power of a Citizen Patient to make it happen. This book is more than a primer in that regard; it's a manual.

This is not an argument for denigrating the physician or the profession of medicine. In every fiber of my being, I believe such would be a great tragedy. It is an argument for the physician and the medical profession to assume an enlightened and enlightening role in contemporary society, one that is based on knowledge as to the limits of certainty and a proclivity to negotiate options with a given patient whenever those limits are exceeded. It is a call for medicine to be truly a service profession because, finally, it is in a position to eschew self-service. It is a call for a transitioning of the "clinic" from a fearful space to a comforting and light-filled space. It is a call for placing any illness, predicament, or anxiety in the broad context of the course of life rather than reduce it only to its most proximate cause and effect. It is a call for Citizen Patients to understand these goals and make them their own.

The Art of Medicine

Physicians have reveled in the phrase "the art of medicine" since antiquity. It has a stately ring, connoting a higher station among life pursuits. It's as though physicians could create something of meaning, even beauty, where there was none before. Composers can do this, painters can, sculptors can . . . but can physicians? We don't speak of priests, lawyers, social workers, or business managers as practicing an art form. Can a physician fashion something original and artful out of the patient-physician interaction? The physician can deduce the cause of illness. The physician can prescribe specific treatments with certain efficacy. Occasionally, the physician can cure. But these are exercises in the science of medicine. The "art" hovers above and beyond the valid diagnosis, effective treatment, and cure.

Art is more than creating something aesthetically pleasing from nothing. Art instructs us in seeing, hearing, and feeling the aesthetic we ignored or missed or that was beyond our sensibilities. All aesthetics are socially constructed. To be an art form, or artful, or beautiful requires recruiting others to consensus. It is hard to imagine that the mid-nineteenth-century audience that applauded opera in Italy would appreciate Noh in contemporaneous Japan—and vice versa. Furthermore, aesthetics are as ephemeral as the consensus that declared something an art. Can medicine be an art in this context? Medicine's science has changed, evolved over the course of millennia by shedding false premises. Medicine's claim to being an art form has no such evolution.

The constant in the patient-physician interaction over the millennia is not the physician's skill in ministering to the ill; that marker is complicated, even to this day. The constant is the paternalistic nature of the physician-patient interaction. Declaring that relationship a thing of beauty, an art form, is testimony to hubris and the inequitable distribution of power. Finally, in the twenty-first century, we have recognized this asymmetry. The suggested "fix," however, is to replace "medicine is an art" with technologies and technologists that fix the fixable. To value the physician mainly for what is done to the patient is no better than what it replaces.

In truth, the physician has never been the artist in the physician-patient relationship; but neither was the patient the canvas. It should be just the opposite: medicine creates the palette and, ideally, the patient has the brush. The physician can explain why a particular hue is more or less appropriate to serve the outcome the patient desires, and why some options are off the palette. But the patient should assume some responsibility for the beauty of the outcome. In such a relationship, the omission of a color or a brush stroke can be as important as what is done.

This principle of patient empowerment can be misinterpreted, even overstated. Patient preferences, preconceptions, and prejudices are always part of the experience of illness, just as they are part of the experience of health. The physician must not only respect this human attribute but also realize how important it is to harness these proclivities to the benefit of the patient when they are reasonable and to disabuse the patient of them when they are unreasonable. In the twenty-first century, medicine should be philosophy: informed by science and imbued with all that is humanity. The practice of medicine is not the reason for medicine to exist, nor is the enshrinement of the practitioner. Medicine's primary calling today is to the personal, unique, idiosyncratic need of each person who chooses to be a patient. No patient should ever again ask, "Doc, what would you do?" Every patient should learn to ask, and be empowered to ask, "Doc, what would you do if you were me?"

Professionalism

This second question has profound implications. It calls for much more than the exercise of the science of medicine: What do you do? What is done? What can be done? It calls for the clinical judgment that can meld the few scientific certainties and the many clinical uncertainties into options that serve the needs of the patient—the one individual who is entitled to the wherewithal to make whatever decision is most suitable. The provision of this clinical judgment should be the physician's role. There is no other reason to seek out the ministrations of a practitioner of medicine. What follows after this exercise—usually treatment—demands skill sets that are far more predictable and often easily delegated. The first decision is intellectually demanding and often value laden; the doing that follows is far more concrete and reproducible. Clinical judgment is the service that renders medicine a profession. The degree to which the delivery of this service is excellent is the degree to which medicine is valuable to society and valued by the individual patient. We should expect no less.

Clinical judgment is both an intellectual exercise and an intimate collaboration. We will have more to say about the former shortly. It is the latter that is underrecognized. If the collaboration is not successful, disquiet and dissatisfaction on the part of the patient can ensue, leading to inappropriate interventions and disappointing outcomes. There can be no intimate clinical collaboration without trust. And trust is a two-way street. The patient must feel secure that the physician is doing everything possible to place her interests above all else.

That is never a trivial demand. The physician must subjugate all pre-conceptions, all emotional responses, and all that might be conflictual to the demands of the collaboration. The physician demeanor must project empathy, promote communication, and encourage confidence. The essence of professionalism is a composite of rigorous competence and trustworthiness that engenders confidence. Other trappings follow naturally: wearing acceptable attire, using appropriate body language, avoiding vernacular, maintaining proper physical distance, smiling, and being prompt.

The last is one bane of being a patient. No one should have to wait beyond the appointed time. Sometimes this is systemic; the organizational infrastructure of the practice setting is a mess. That's inexcusable. Sometimes an unexpected, infuriating delay is unavoidable. After all, much of clinical medicine is unpredictable. If your own clinical interview calls for actions and behaviors that consumed unexpected time, you would not appreciate someone telling you, "Time's up." It takes little time, though, for the physician or staff to keep you abreast of the reasons for delay and to offer you options. That's not just courtesy; that's part of the intimate collaboration that is the reason you sought care in the first place.

In return for professionalism, it is necessary for the patient to participate to the fullest possible extent in the exercise of clinical judgment so that its goal can be realized. The goal is to enable the patient to assume responsibility for making clinical decisions by informed choice. There is no other goal. This is an intimate clinical collaboration, not a friendship. In fact, it is not necessary for the physician to "like" the patient to maintain professionalism. Nor is it necessary for the patient to "like" the physician. To the contrary, emotional distance promotes objectivity on both parts. "Friendship" and stronger emotional bonding between patient and physician have no role to play in the collaboration. In fact, they can be very intrusive and counterproductive; in such cases, both parties should call for a substitute physician rather than risk a distortion in clinical judgment.

Clinical Judgment Is Not Adjudicatory

Let's get real: this two-way street can be rutted. There are streets where the rutting is predictable. One such situation is when the physician is performing as a gatekeeper, particularly in the context of disability determination. In these sorts of interactions, the physician is contracted by a third party to sit in judgment of, or even to question aggressively, the patient's complaints. The patient is forewarned when entering such a relationship. This is not a therapeutic encounter: it can be Kafkaesque. I have argued for decades that physicians who participate in such a tribunal are behaving not as physicians but as agents of the state. There is no valid science they can bring to this circumstance, and their preconceptions are no more informed than those of the laity. (I discuss this in detail in *Stabbed in the Back*.)

If this is your fate, at least appreciate the rules of engagement. These encounters have nothing in common with the "intimate clinical collaboration" we've been discussing. I have been advocating removing disability determination and other forms of gatekeeping from the medical arena. Unfortunately, this is an aspect of life that escapes the attention of those not involved and that is a source of income for many who are involved in the gatekeeping, from physicians and lawyers to the insurance industry. Only the claimants suffer mightily. Clinical judgment and gatekeeping are incompatible roles.

Another circumstance in which the two-way street is always rutted is not a legal construct but a social construct. There are individuals who are ill, often pervasively ill, but for whom the science of medicine can find little that is not "normal." All our testing has failed to produce a specific diagnosis. That's a dreadful circumstance in our culture, which demands that illness be diagnosed first before coping can proceed. Rather than being reassured by the "negative" workup, these individuals find themselves confronted with and affronted by the imprecation, "Could it be in your mind?" This query is reasonable, but it is a semiotic that connotes weakness, feigning, even malingering.

The result is that these sufferers feel beleaguered, angry, and defensive and bring all these emotions to any "intimate clinical collaboration." Their narrative of illness is laced with idioms that reflect a combination of desperation and defensiveness. Most physicians sense this and bristle, which further heightens the patient's antipathy. In such a circumstance, trust is impossible. So, too, is healing, as no one can start to feel better if they have to prove they are ill.

Some physicians are comfortable supporting these patients under the banner: "There is no possibility that this is in your mind. Someday we will know the cause." Other physicians bandy descriptive labels for diagnoses, many of which are neologisms like fibromyalgia, chronic fatigue syndrome, temporomandibular joint syndrome, and irritable bowel syndrome that lend themselves to facile acronyms: FM, CFS, TMJ, IBS, etc. Of course, all are merely reiterations of the chief complaint or the complaint that the diagnostician is most comfortable hearing. These sufferers generally express a panoply of symptoms that qualify them for more than one label. They are most comfortable under the care of sectarian physicians who do such labeling, although their prognosis in terms of being able to assert "I'm well again" is still dismal.

I wish we could change the social construction that draws these ill individuals into this vortex. I wish I would see a time when a patient went before a physician with some variation of the complaint mentioned in chapter 6: "I feel awful. Could it be in my mind?" Then the physician could respond by saying that "in your mind" is a lot better than many alternatives. Today, no such repartee is possible. Alas. I discuss this phenomenology in detail in *Stabbed in the Back* and, before that, in *Worried Sick*.

Clinical judgment in the service of patients with somatoform disorders is sorely tested and begs circumspection at the very least. All of these patients enter the clinic with the same goal as any other patient: to find out what is causing their distress and to have the cause remedied. Many would be relieved with an answer that should be distressful, such as multiple sclerosis. They find such a label a relief, a "now I know" event. No one likes uncertainty. But these patients are not likely to feel satisfied if they are spared labeling. "I don't know" will drive them on to seek an answer elsewhere. Most are aware of the somatoform labels and acronyms and are either already labeled or predisposed to being labeled in this fashion. They are likely to be angry if the clinician is uncomfortable doing so. No one is nurtured by such an interaction.

The establishment of a trusting, collaborative relationship is not unique to medical professionalism. All professionalism demands as much. Without such a relationship, we'd all find another attorney, or dentist, or clergy, or . . . . For some professions, the trusting relationship is part of the treatment act itself. That is certainly true of medical professionalism. People feel better and are more likely to anticipate further improvement at the hands of and/or in the presence of another person who is trusted. As Martin Buber so eloquently wrote in *The Knowledge of Man*:

> Man wishes to be confirmed in his being by man,
> and wishes to have a presence in the being of the other. . . .
> Secretly and bashfully he watches for a YES which allows him
> to be and which can come only from one human person to another.

Professionalism and the Contemporary Institution of Medicine

Many forces vie for entry into the clinic, including forces that threaten clinical judgment. Some relate to cross-purposes between patient and physician, such as is inherent in caring for and about patients with somatoform disorders and in gatekeeper functions. Many more are a result of conflicts of interest on the part of the physician. The most discussed of these are personal acts on the part of the physician, some intentional and others subliminal, that need not, or do not, serve the best interests of the patient. The most obvious relate to the fine line between marketing and bribery walked by the pharmaceutical and medical-device industries. These were dissected in detail in earlier chapters.

There has always been at least as great a risk, however, of self-serving behaviors inherent in the structure of any profession, and medicine is no exception. For all that is good in the history of professional credentialing and peer review, there is much that is bad. Traditionally, this soft underbelly of professionalism relates to the degree professions are a throwback to medieval guilds that aggressively staked out their turf, guarded their monopoly, and maximized their profitability. The guilds grew in power and self-aggrandizement; they became an end in and of themselves. To accomplish this required, and still requires, a pecking order among the professionals. This is an exercise in group psychology in which attributes termed "leadership" come into play, attributes that may have little or nothing to do with professional competence and clinical judgment. Just as in other aspects of life in which individuality is subjugated to the success of the group, leadership is succored by elements that fuel its own power. Enlightened and progressive leadership is a special accident. More typically, leadership accumulates power by recruiting sycophants rather than by farsightedness or the setting of standards of professional competence by example. Bridling power for power's sake is realpolitik. To some degree, we all learned this in grade school.

Today, we no longer talk of a guild in the medieval sense. We are more comfortable with the tautology the "institution" of medicine. In the mid-twentieth century, the American Medical Association was the organizational embodiment of the institution of medicine. This monolith has since been balkanized; specialty and subspecialty organizations create cacophony. What is less appreciated is that over the course of the past fifty years, the polyglot institution of medicine is no longer modulated by realpolitik; it is subsumed. The institution of medicine takes marching orders from lay organizations as to how the clinic is to be organized, how clinical judgment is to be utilized, how all is underwritten, who is eminent, and who leads. The conflicts of interest for which the institution of medicine is but a front reflect the agendas of multiple nongovernmental and governmental organizations.

The burden on the Citizen Patient is compounded as a result. Not only must one be wary of personal conflicts of interest on the part of the physician, but one also must be wary of the conflicts of interest on the part of institutions to which the physician is responsive if not beholden. Physicians in the twenty-first century are increasingly likely to be working for organizations whose leadership and funding are ever more distant from the clinic and whose agendas are ever more foreign to clinical judgment. Nearly all such organizations have Orwellian monikers, such as "patient-centered," "accountable," and "medical home." All of these have in common the notion that patients are better off if as many elements of care as possible, and their coordination, are delegated so that performance is efficient and cost is contained. All of them take as a given that technically demanding interventions are necessary, and necessarily costly, sacred cows. All take as a given that the tried is true and can be taken for granted as cost-effective. For all these organizations, the challenge of "health-care" delivery is in the appropriate distribution of all the latest, newest, fanciest, most costly, and most profitable procedure, pharmaceutical, or widget.

Clinical judgment barely gets lip service in this formulation. That's disconcerting, since without clinical judgment, the formulation is terribly flawed. Patients become "units of care" looked after by providers who are rewarded for "throughput." It's an efficient way to get your blood pressure and blood sugar "monitored" but not a way for you to question the degree to which the monitoring advantages you—the aspect of the treatment that is far more critical than any other from your perspective. Clinical judgment and retailing have absolutely nothing in common. Caveat emptor works with retailing because we won't buy a lemon twice. When it comes to the provision of health care, though, the patient is likely to be blamed for the bad outcome.

Clinical judgment needs effective championing, which can come only from Citizen Patients who see clearly through all the self-interest and want to trust that their physician will respond to "What would you do if you were me?" with the undivided attention, competence, and trustworthiness the query deserves.

Evidence-Based Medicine

Every profession has specialized expertise, a body of knowledge that is brought to the trusting relationship and for which the professional is sought out. The medical profession touts science as its special asset and, when science is lacking, falls back on the same cushions arrayed by every other profession: experience and peer review. All of this begs transparency and reflection.

Someday, soon I hope, it will be reasonable for a patient to assume that the conversation with a physician is truly informed by the state of the science. For reasons that were emphasized throughout this book, that assumption is wrong far too often. Therefore, the patient must approach all options under consideration with an ear toward the evidentiary basis for acceptance. Has the option been studied systematically in patients similar to me and with a similar indication for intervening? If so, how compelling is the evidence that I am more likely to be helped than harmed? If I am more likely to be helped than harmed, to what degree will I be helped? These are queries that are the foundation of the age of "evidence-based medicine" (EBM), an age that arrived at full bloom only in the past decade or two in response to the size and scope of the international efforts in clinical investigation.

Tens of thousands of clinical investigations are undertaken each year. They vary in their purview and in their scientific rigor. Even academicians such as me are hard-pressed to keep up with literatures out of the mainstream, and increasingly hard-pressed with the mainstream literature in the several disciplines in which I purport "expertise." There is always the concern that I am overlooking something crucial, or that, despite my training and proclivities, I am swayed by shoddy science.

In response to this quandary, a new science has evolved dedicated to reviewing the literature, separating the wheat from the chaff, and identifying the most delectable of kernels. There is now a substantial international effort to this end. Literally thousands of investigators have been recruited to the task, and systematic reviews of various aspects of the clinical literature abound. As a result, no longer is there just an enormous literature to review; there is also a growing literature about the literature to review. Furthermore, each reviewer brings preconceptions to the task. After all, this is a clinical literature, not nuclear physics. There is always room for debate as to the quality of any given study and the sway it should have on clinical decision making. One reviewer can forgive as minor the same methodological weakness another considers critical. Systematic reviews of studies of the efficacy of a particular drug on a particular disease can vary dramatically. For example, systematic reviews sponsored by industry are far more likely to deem the sponsor's drug efficacious than systematic reviews of the same literature sponsored by governments.

On this background, several agencies have come into being dedicated to sifting the medical literature with as little prejudice as possible. The godfather of this movement is the Cochrane Database of Systematic Reviews, introduced in chapter 6. These are resources that inform medical decision making but do not substitute for the exercise of clinical judgment in the course of an intimate clinical collaboration. It turns out that the vast majority of the clinical literature is so lacking in methodological quality as to offer no contribution of substance to clinical decision making. For most clinical questions, one is fortunate to find a dozen studies that can be deemed informative. These studies often vary in the definition of the outcome they study and in the types of patients they recruit as subjects. Such variability challenges attempts to identify reproducibility between studies, and reproducibility is the most reassuring attribute of any scientific result. For many clinical interventions, the science fails to demonstrate any efficacy. Many of the studies that demonstrate the efficacy of a particular intervention differ in the degree to which the intervention proved efficacious. Much more often than not, the magnitude of clinical effect is underwhelming. The result is that for many an instance of EBM, the most that can be asserted with confidence is that the evidence for benefit is lacking despite valiant attempts to demonstrate benefit in particular kinds of patients. Occasionally, one can assert that there is evidence for benefit in a particular patient population but the effect is so small that the result is tenuous. That means that the evidence to sway the decision to accept or reject much that is available and much that is commonly prescribed is flimsy. Where does that leave clinical judgment? One answer is to ask why so many interventions are available for use despite a science that supports an assertion of inefficacy or minimal efficacy. That's a great question, one that is central to our considerations in this book. Another answer is a dialogue between patient and physician regarding whether and how such flimsy evidence might be parsed to the particular patient's advantage.

Clinical Experience and Peer Review

Now we are ready to consider the corollary query, "What would you do if you were me and there was no compelling science to inform the decision?" The answer is that we would rely on clinical judgment. This is "clinical judgment" in its finest hour, when it must rely solely on the degree to which wisdom can grow from the trusting collaboration between a particular physician and a particular patient. Clinical judgment is anchored in the circumstances that are unique to the particular patient; it does not take refuge in a determinative literature or the clinician's preconceived notions. I have been told that I have great "clinical judgment" throughout my career and have been selected for most of the "best doctors" lists in testimony to my reputation. But I have been practicing for forty years. I can tell you that much that is lauded as clinical judgment stands the test of time poorly. It is quite humbling. But if it is a collaborative event, it may be the best available at the time the patient is ill; the doctor and the patient are in it together.

To be an excellent clinician and clinical scholar demands a lifetime of continuing medical education (CME). For the reasons discussed above regarding the limitations of evidence-based medicine, however, the scientific advance of this year is likely to be superseded by the advance of next year, including the advance that finds its forerunner lacking. Besides, there are many clinical issues and challenges about which there is no informative science, and many that are so idiosyncratic as to preclude the possibility of clinical science.

Truth be told, such circumstances are still more frequent than medicine is wont to admit or the public is comfortable learning. In fact, such circumstances are the rule for the "cognitive specialties," where little if anything is done *to* the patient while as much as is suitable is done *for* the patient. The traditional fallback in determining what is suitable is to turn away from the bedside, then draw on one's clinical experience and collect the input of peers before returning to the bedside with an awesome display of "clinical judgment." This is the essence of "What would you do, Doc?," instead of "What would you do if you were me?" It is the form of clinical judgment that should not be carried forward into the twenty-first century. It is not tried and true; to the contrary, all too often it is tried and false. The "clinical judgment" that is the sole purview of the clinician is at the mercy of the foibles of clinical experience and of peer review. And foibles abound.

Clinical experience is the accumulation of clinical anecdotes. It is assumed that the input and the recall are valued objectively based on an appreciation of patient outcomes. That is not a valid assumption. All such recall is telescoped; we are likely to remember the more recent events. More important, the more dramatic events are harder to forget. If a patient suffers an unexpected and rare fatal event, clinical experience is disturbed; the clinician is far more likely to fear such an event in the next patient with a similar presentation. Likewise, if clinical experiences are consistently favorable in a particular circumstance, clinicians are likely to let their guards down.

And then there's the pitfall of the "good idea." In contemporary culture, the pressure is to "don't just stand there, do something!" This is usually dressed up as "empirical therapy," a form of "let's see if this works." Usually there is a rationale, but by definition, the rationale of empirical therapy is untested. Many a patient has received antibiotics or chemotherapy as empirical therapies. Of course, these agents are available, having been licensed for particular indications based on a science that convinced the FDA as to efficacy. But the contemporary clinical ethos countenances "off-label" use as empirical therapy. Empirical therapies have a great tendency to become rooted in "clinical experience." If one patient does well, even if that is but a coincidence, it's hard for a clinician not to return to the same empirical therapy in a similar clinical circumstance. Unfortunately, if the patient does poorly, it's hard for a clinician to leap to the conclusion that the therapy was a dumb thing to do; it's far easier to bemoan the intransigent nature of the patient's disease. "Clinical experience" is an important element of the collaboration between a patient and a physician, but it should not be determinative.

Peer review is another important aspect of the clinician's input into informed medical decision making. Peer review is a tenet of professionalism, regardless of the profession. All physicians should be able to display and defend their care of a patient before their peers and should feel compelled to do so. "What am I missing?" and "What more could I do?" are noble questions, not admissions of inadequacy. They are also not integral to the "intimate clinical collaboration" because their answering does not demand the patient-physician bond of trust, only a physician-physician bond of trust. But they offer much-needed reassurance in the setting of clinical uncertainty.

Unfortunately, peer review is highly imperfect. First of all, peers are peers because they are of like mind. They wear the same rose-colored glasses. Therein lies the folly of peer review, whether it's convened for the sake of the care of a patient or for the sake of scientific publication. The fate of a peer with a divergent opinion is predictable: to borrow the Japanese proverb *Deru kugi wa utareru*, the nail that sticks out gets hammered down. It's far easier for peers to argue who does something better than to question whether that thing should be done at all.

Peer review can only illuminate when there is an element of controversy in an atmosphere of collegiality. For those of us who grew up in the American era of clinical scholarship, controversy was as valued as collegiality. There were weekly meetings, often called "Morbidity and Mortality Conferences," where clinicians would examine the machinations of peers from the distance of the clinical records, looking for errors in commission and omission and arguing whether there was or is a better way. Students would attend in awe. Tempers were allowed to flare as long as the interchanges were constructive. The limits of certainty were defined and thereby the need for additional information became evident. The ethic of peer review became so entrenched that the need for constructive controversy moved to real time and active decision making. Consultants would do battle in conference rooms near the bedsides of patients whose future was at stake. The defeat of the consultant was not to be personalized; this was not to be an exercise in the power of personality but in the degree to which science and clinical experience were inadequate. All levels of students were recruited to these exercises to experience clinical scholarship as a lifestyle.

There is barely a vestige of this activity left in American hospitals. Clinical disciplines are compartmentalized, creating isolated peer groups. Defining the limits of certainty is no longer vaunted. It is too time-consuming and has been subjugated to "throughput," or managing the case so as to maximize cash flow. "Morbidity and Mortality Rounds" have become abstract discussions of potential hazards so as not to expose the clinicians and the institute to the risk of malpractice suits, which might arise if these rounds were still clinical object lessons. Peer review, always a tenuous exercise, has become a euphemism. The country learned this when the dim lights leading the insurance industry introduced the notion of a compulsory second opinion for expensive procedures. That proved a waste of time and money. The American counter to the Japanese proverb is that if you have a hammer, everything looks like a nail. If your physician seeks peer review on your behalf and not in the service of another agenda, applause and gratitude are called for.

"Cognitive Specialties"

I introduced the term "cognitive specialty" above in quotation marks. This rubric is not my invention. It is used by many as the designation for clinical specialties that do not require competence in physical interventions, surgical interventions especially. The cognitive specialties demand reflection and cognition rather than technical prowess. I have been certified by American boards in internal medicine, rheumatology, allergy and immunology, and geriatrics and admitted to fellowship in occupational medicine. All of these are "cognitive specialties." I am proud to count myself among the practitioners of the cognitive specialties. However, the rubric has always engendered cognitive dissonance for me. What are the noncognitive specialists practicing? Are they mindless technocrats? Of course not—although some of their procedures require little skill and others more perseverance than skill (think colonoscopy). "Cognitive specialists" is a label for practitioners who for their efforts at thoughtfulness are reimbursed less than are interventionalists for performing procedures.

A term such as "cognitive specialty" did not gain a foothold because it made sense. It followed from a dramatic semiotic shift that occurred after World War II. In keeping with the aphorism generally attributed to Hippocrates, "First, do no harm" (*primum non nocere*), medicine long gave lip service to "conservative care." Clinical judgment called for that which was cautious and familiar. In antiquity, the inventive physician prone to empirical therapies was looked down upon. In ancient Greece, an empiric was a quack.

In the 1960s, advances in anesthesia and in surgery improved the safety of both, and so surgical inventiveness was unleashed. Surgical technology made great leaps forward, and it continues to do so today. The first wave of advances allowed surgeons to manipulate the cardiovascular structures in ways never before possible. We are now witnessing the second wave because technology has facilitated approaching all sorts of disease with small instruments through small portals of entry. It is all being done quicker, with less trauma and fewer complications. These dramatic technological advances are worthy of the awe engendered by a medical press that breathlessly covers every nuance. But this awe has evolved into a cultlike belief in the technological solutions to human dilemmas and a tendency to value them without question. One manifestation of this irrational love of interventions is the willingness to accept escalating costliness for anything that is interventional. This is across the board. A dermatologist can be reimbursed $250 for cutting off a wart in a minute or two but only $30 for monitoring the therapeutic response of a patient with psoriasis. Today, "conservative" care is no longer reasonable and cautious; it's nihilism. Whereas "aggressive" care is valued indiscriminately and absurdly cost accounted.

Citizen Patients need to understand this dialectic and decry its excesses, both in the halls of policy and, more urgently, at their own bedside. There is no such thing as a "cognitive specialty"; the profession of medicine is a cognitive exercise. As for being in awe of technology or cowed by the putative skillfulness it requires: caveat emptor. The principles of informed medical decision making are inviolate. They pertain when the intervention is no more dramatic than dialogue. The mandate to establish a trusting collaborative relationship remains primary.

Continuing Medical Education

We discussed above the fashion in which the agendas of the institution of medicine can be inserted into the clinic, placing constraints on clinical judgment that shade to the unethical. In an earlier chapter, we discussed also the responsibility of the individual physician to avoid personal conflicts of interest. There is a little-appreciated arena in which both personal and institutional agendas assault the ethical foundation of clinical judgment. That arena is the form that continuing medical education takes in the institutions that most doctors practice in.

I stated above, "To be an excellent clinician and clinical scholar demands a lifetime of continuing medical education." That assertion is codified: all states require documentation as to CME for licensure and relicensure. The CME I discussed above relates to reading the literature and engaging in peer review. However, CME is an industry in American medicine and in many other licensed professional groups. Everyone has to attend a certain number of hours of costly formal education, usually in something approaching a lecture format. There are studies demonstrating the marginal retention of information following CME. There are also studies documenting the conflictual nature of medical continuing education where CME has a marketing agenda. Legitimate peer review and responsive professionalism are no longer considered adequate because they are difficult to quantify and even more difficult to corrupt. I have watched this evolution with vociferous disgust.

When I joined the faculty at the University of North Carolina at Chapel Hill forty years ago, there were few rheumatologists in North Carolina. I proposed to the person in the dean's office responsible for CME that we serve the state's physicians by holding an annual rheumatology update. He was encouraging, but he suggested that I forgo the notion of a tuition-free session. He said that "if you don't charge, docs undervalue the exercise and don't attend." We charged a pittance and held well-attended, highly interactive sessions for several years, until our down-home efforts were superseded by the iron grip of the CME industry. Within a decade, I understood that CME was engulfed in an ever-more-sophisticated marketing exercise benefiting all sorts of stakeholders. I have eschewed any role in this enterprise ever since, from speakers' bureaus to free anything. In addition to reading the literature, I am inclined to real-time CME. I write long, often didactic letters to doctors who refer patients to me and spend much time conferring with colleagues regarding particularly challenging cases. We learn piecemeal, but we learn.

I firmly believe that interactive peer learning is a pillar of the medical profession and other professions. There is no expert worth his salt who doesn't need to gain in expertise. There is no specialist whose purview is so constrained that considering uncertainties outside that discipline is irrelevant; even patients of ophthalmologists have hearts and joints. We all need CME enriched by peers with special perspectives and knowledge. "Keeping up" is not optional; our patients trust us to do so, and we are morally committed to it as physicians.

There must be a way to make the peer learning experience efficient without compromising its sole rationale: the continuing improvement of the quality of the care we afford our patients. None of us should have to wonder if the expert is actually hawking a drug, procedure, or widget. And none of us is so financially stressed that he or she needs a free meal or a briefcase with a logo.

Our "teachers" must consider teaching as much a moral obligation as do their peers who come to question and learn. Since "students" bring to the exercise experiences and perspectives that facilitate active and interactive learning, any fee for educational services goes both ways and cancels out. Hence, the expense of peer-based CME should be minimal.

I envision a system of live Web seminars held frequently at every medical school. A few expert conveners and a dozen physician learners sit around a table discussing a topic. Anyone can register to listen in, even to submit queries beforehand. Links on the website can take any participant directly to the primary references and supplemental readings. Since we live in a country of bean counters, the registering "counts"—but it is the learning that matters.

The stumbling block to such a simple change in the concept of CME would surprise the laity, but not those of us who understand the ethical lapses that plague the American institution of medicine. The work of medical schools is barely discernible in the academic health centers, and medical education is a cost center. Academic health centers are non-profit corporations with market agendas as crass as any we denounce. Too often, clinical thought leaders are hired to create profit centers; marketing their latest technique, regimen, or gizmo is requisite to competing with profit centers in neighboring academic institutions. Can the academic rheumatologist or oncologist speak about biologic and other drugs without the infusion clinic's spreadsheet looming, at least subliminally? Can the cardiologist look objectively at the door-to-catheter data without considering the volume of his own catheterization lab? The only protections against ethical blind spots are from peers at the seminar table who are duty bound to hold all assertions up to the clear light of day. If my colleagues want a reunion with like-minded physicians or a networking event on the golf course of some resort, they can go ahead—but they, and not their fellow taxpayers or someone trying to buy their approach to patient care, should pay for it. And if they want a speaker or entertainment, that, too, should be on their nickel.

Conclusion

QUO VADIS

Well, my dear Citizen Patient, the ball is in your court. You, en masse, have the power to confront the status quo despite its very deep pockets and minions of lobbyists committed to the preservation of the stakes held by the stakeholders. You can cry foul and be heard, even across the barriers built to buffer our elected officials. You can point your collective fingers at every individual perverse aspect of the current American "health-care system." You can even generate rallying cries such as, "Give me the Canadian—or French, Dutch, British, German, Finnish, Israeli—system, or bust!" I will applaud. I will join your march. I'm much happier as your pamphleteer than in your vanguard. But I will do my best.

We are likely to fail. The American health-care system is as entrenched and wealthy as it is perverse. It is also clearly unsustainable. It is hell-bent for collapse, and its leadership is much more committed to and adept at self-service than it is farsighted or ethical. The result will be turbulent, and many a lovely servant to the ill and many an ill patient will be sorely served during this time.

But this will pass, and there will be time for reflection. That's when you need to speak out. If I'm still alive, you can count on my voice. You know what sort of phoenix you want to emerge.

Index

Page numbers in *italics* refer to figures and tables.

Absolute frequencies, 86–87

Academic health centers: administration of, 14, *16–17, 18*; competition for patients among, 14, 23–24; conflicts of interest at, 6, 9–10, 13, 221; Contract Research Organizations created by, 24, 189; in escalation of health-care costs, 47–51; marketing by, 19–21, 221; medical education at, 6, 221; mission of, 14–15; origins and rise of, 47–51; rankings of, 23

ACP Journal Club, 185, 195

Acronyms, 171, 172, 210

Active-active trials, 148, 150

Acupuncture, 150, 156

ADD, 177

Administrative costs: in Disease Insurance–Health Assurance approach, 198; facility fees to cover, 15; per capita, international comparison of, 181. *See also* Hospital administration

Adrenaline, 61

Advanced Science and Technology Adjudication Resource (ASTAR) Program, 94–95

Adverse effects: in randomized controlled trials, 186, 187; reporting of, to FDA, 31

Advertising. *See* Marketing

Advocacy groups, disease-specific, 34–36

Aesthetics, 206

Aetna, 55, 56

Affective disorders, placebo effect in, 152

Affordable Care Act of 2010, 55, 178–79

Agency for Healthcare Research and Quality (AHRQ), 41

Alcohol: consumption of, and longevity, 119–23, *122*; metabolism of, genetics in, 140

Allied health professionals, in clinics in retail stores, 204

Alternative theories, 72–73

American Association of Medical Colleges, 11, 12–13

American Cancer Foundation, 36

American Cancer Society (ACS), 35–36

American College of Physicians, 185

American College of Rheumatology (ACR), 35, 174

American Heart Association (AHA), 34–35

American Home, 60

American Hospital Association, 55

American Institutes for Research, 167

American Journal of Public Health, 126

American Medical Association (AMA): balkanization of, 211; on chiropractic, 166; Code of Medical Ethics of, 64, 166, 200–201; Current Procedural Terminology of, 65; in origins of Medicare, 45; in setting of fee structure, 45, 46, 67–68, 200–201

American Petroleum Institute, 132

American Recovery and Reinvestment Act of 2009, 74

American Rheumatism Association (ARA), 35, 174

American Society for the Control of Cancer (ASCC), 35. *See also* American Cancer Society

Amgen, 36

Amitriptyline, 156

Anderson Cancer Center, 142

Angina: advances in understanding of, 88; treatment of, 88, 89, 99–102, 150–51

Angioplasty: *vs.* CABG, 98, 99; development of, 97–98; efficacy of, 95–101; trials of, 98–99; as Type II Medical Malpractice, 118

Animal magnetism, 149

Animal research, 21, 25

Ankylosing spondylitis, 140

Annals of Internal Medicine, 21

Annual examinations, 197

Antibiotics, development of, 60–61

Antidepressants, tricyclic, 174

Archives of Internal Medicine, 113

Arm pain, placebo effect in, 156

Army, U.S., 112

Arthritis: cost of treatment of, 42, *42*, *43*; disease foundations dedicated to, 35. *See also* Rheumatoid arthritis

Arthritis Foundation (AF), 35

Arthroscopy, knee, 108–9

Art of medicine, 205–7

Asperger's syndrome, 177

Aspirin, 59–60, 87

Association of Health Care Journalists, 20, 21

Asthma, 161

AstraZeneca, marketing by, 36–40

Astrology, 84

Atheism, 158

Atherosclerosis, definition of, 88. *See also* Coronary artery disease

Atrazine, 134

Austin, Peter, 84

Authors, conflicts of interest in, 11

Average responses, in randomized controlled trials, 79–80

Avicenna, 73

Baby aspirin, 87

Back pain: coping with, 129–30; cost of treatment of, 42, *42*, *43*; placebo effect in, 152; subjectivity in experience of, 148; trials of surgical interventions for, 187–88; ubiquity of, 129–30; workers' compensation claims for, 57, 129–30

Bacon, Francis, 158

BARI-2D trial, 99

Barker, Kristin, 172, 177

Bayer aspirin, 60

Baylor University, 55

Beecher, Henry, 149–50

Bendectin, 92

Benefit/harm, in comparative effectiveness research, 75, 76

Bennett, James T., 36

Benzene, 132–33

Berkman, Lisa, 125

Berryhill, Reece, *181*

Berry Plan, 49

Bias. *See* Conflicts of interest; Ethics

Billing for health care: coding in, 65–66, 201; DRG-based, 65–66; history of, 65; at hospitals, 65–67; on sliding scale, 64, 201. *See also* Costs of health care

Biology, of poverty, 128–29

Biopsychosocial model of illness, 168, 169

Biostatistics, history of, 123–24

Birth of the Clinic, The (Foucault), 204–5

Black, James, 61, 62

Blockbuster drugs, 62–63

Blood pressure, high. *See* Hypertension

Blood sugar, high, treatment of, 81–82

Blue Cross Association, 55

Blue Cross Blue Shield Association (BCBS), 55, 56

Blue Shield plans, 55

Bonds, municipal, 14, 53

Bone mineral density, 135

BPA, 134

Bradshaw, John, 62

Brain, 169–70. *See also* Mind

BRCA-1 gene, 137–38; BRCA-2 gene, 137–38

Breast cancer: genetics of, 137–38; screening for (*See* Mammography); tumor-specific chemotherapeutic agents for, 141

Brigham Hospital, 40, 156

Bristol-Myers, 60

Britain: life-course epidemiology in, 125; pharmaceutical industry in, 61–62; poverty and longevity in, 128

British Medical Journal, 156, 167

Buber, Martin, 210

Bubonic plague, 145–46

Bull Moose Party, 182, 200

Burroughs-Wellcome, 25, 61, 62, 190

Bush, George H. W., 67

Business model(s): of hospitals, 23–24; of insurance industry, 191–92; of pharmaceutical industry, 189

Business Week, 100

CABG. *See* Coronary artery bypass graft surgery

California, origins of insurance in, 55

Canada, health-care costs in, 181

Cancer: cost of treatment of, 42, *42*, *43*; disease foundations dedicated to, 35–36; genetics of, 137–38, 140–42; imaging techniques for, 146; ionizing radiation and, 111, 113–14, *114*; off-label use of drugs for, 31; pharmacogenetics in treatment of, 140–42; stages of, 146; Type II Medical Malpractice in, 118; war on, 35. *See also specific types*

Canon of Medicine, The (Avicenna), 73

Capitalism, job satisfaction and longevity in, 131

Cardiac catheterization, 88, 89, 101–2

Cardiology, disease foundations dedicated to, 34–35. *See also* Interventional cardiology

Cardiovascular disease, risk factors for, 125–26. *See also* Coronary artery disease

Care of Strangers, The (Rosenberg), 51

Carey, John, 100

Carman, Kristin, 167

Case-control studies, 184

CAT. *See* Computerized tomography

Catastrophizing, 165, 171, 173

Catheterization, cardiac, 88, 89, 101–2

CDC. *See* Centers for Disease Control

Cement, 151–52

Center for Devices and Radiologic Health, FDA, 103–4

Centers for Disease Control (CDC), 44, 49

Centers for Medicare and Medicaid Services (CMS), 65–68; conflicts of interest in, 67–68; establishment of physician fees by, 67–68; lack of transparency in, 68; negotiation of costs with hospitals, 67; political pressures on, 192; as self-insurance by federal government, 58; on vertebroplasty coverage, 151, 192

Cervical cancer, screening for, 135

Chain, Ernst, 60

Charities, disease-specific, 34–36

Charity care, 64

Charles (prince of Wales), 167

Chemotherapy, 111, 140–41

Chest pain. *See* Angina

Chiropractic, 157, 165–66

Cholecystectomy, laparoscopic, 105–6

Cholesterol, high: Crestor for treatment of, 36–40; efficacy of treatment of, 80–81; and longevity, 126; screening for, 81, 135, 136

Christian Science, 157

Chronic fatigue syndrome (CFS), 171, 209–10

Churchill, Winston, 60

Cigna, 55, 56, 69

Cimetidine, 61, 62

Class I devices, 103

Class II devices, 103

Class III devices, 103, 104

Clinic(s), 203–21; art of medicine and, 205–7; conflicts of interest in, 6–10, 211–12; future of, 205; history of, 204–5; as meeting of minds *vs.* physical space, 204–5; professionalism in, 207–12; in retail stores, 201; timeliness in, 208. *See also* Clinical judgment

Clinical Center of National Institutes of Health, 48, 49

Clinical interviews: in Disease Insurance–Health Assurance approach, 196–97; importance of, 196

Clinical Journal of the American Society of Nephrology, 81n

Clinical judgment, 207–21; clinical experience in, 215–16; clinical interviews in, 196–97; in cognitive specialties, 215, 218–19; collaboration in, 207–8; conflicts of interest in, 211–12; continuing medical education in, 215, 219–21; in disability determinations, 208–9; as essential role of physicians, 207–8; influence of ran-

domized controlled trials on, 73–74; peer review in, 215–17; reviews of literature in, 213–14

Clinical trials. *See* Trials

Clinimetrics centers, 190, 194–98

Clinton, Bill, 178

Clopidigrel, 98–99, 100

CMS. *See* Centers for Medicare and Medicaid Services

Cochrane Collaboration, 160–61, 160n, 167, 185, 195

Cochrane Database of Systemic Reviews, 214

Coding, medical, 65–66, 201

Cognitive behavioral therapy, 197

Cognitive impairment, screening for, 136

Cognitive specialties, 218–19; clinical judgment in, 215, 218–19; definition of, 218; in fee structures, 46, 68, 218–19; origins of term, 218

Cohort studies, 184

Colchicine, 72

Collaboration, in physician-patient relationship, 204–5, 207–8

Collective conscience, 131

Collins, Francis, 158–59

Colonoscopy, 136, 137, 201

Colorectal cancer: genetics of, 137; screening for, 135, 136, 137

Committee on Comparative Effectiveness Research Prioritization, 74

Common practice, in Disease Insurance–Health Assurance approach, 196–97

Commonwealth Fund, 44, 68–69

Community: definition of, 131; and longevity, 131–32

Comparative effectiveness research (CER), 74–77

Compassionate use of pharmaceutical drugs, 32–33

Compensable back injury, 129

Competition: for patients, 14, 23–24; in scientific process, 12

Complementary medicine, 166–67

Composite outcomes of trials, 28

Computerized decision aids, 196

Computerized tomography (CT or CAT) imaging: of cancer, 146; ionizing radiation in, 112–15, *113*, *114*

Conflicts of interest, 5–40; in academic health centers, 6, 9–10, 13, 221; in clinical setting, 6–10, 211–12; in continuing medical education, 7–9, 13, 219–21; in Contract Research Organizations, 24, 28–29, 40, 63, 189–90; in disease foundations, 35; in employer-based health insurance, 191–92; in FDA drug-approval process, 87; in fee structures, setting of, 67–68; in health-care reform, 189–91; in health journalism, 20–21; institutionalization of, 12–13, 189–90, 211–12; list of problems caused by, 5; in medical literature, 10–12; in pharmaceutical marketing to physicians, 6–10, 211; physician disclosure of, 7–12; in physician relationships with industry, 10; in trials, 24–33, 36–40, 63

Confounders, in relationship between alcohol and longevity, 121–23, *122*

Congress, U.S.: on fibromyalgia, 172; lobbying of, 6, 180, 201; National Institutes of Health renamed by, 48; on pharmaceutical devices, 103; on pharmaceutical marketing to physicians, 6

Connecticut General Life Insurance Company, 55

Consent. *See* Informed consent

Conservative care, 108, 218–19

Consumers, patients as, 91

Continuing medical education (CME), 219–21; in clinical judgment, 215,

219–21; conflicts of interest in, 7–9, 13, 219–21; costs of, 220; interactive peer learning in, 216–17, 220; pharmaceutical marketing in, 7–9, 30; requirements for, 219

Contract Research Organizations (CROs), 24–30; conflicts of interest in, 24, 28–29, 40, 63, 189–90; data analysis by, 28–29; in health-care reform, 188–90; motivations of, 24, 63, 189–90; origins of, 24–25, 63; positive trial outcomes at, 24, 29, 63, 189; recruitment of subjects by, 29–30

Contracts, cost-plus, 19, 57–58

Co-pay, 199

Coping: with back pain, 129–30; in definitions of health, 165, 199; diagnosis as requirement for, 209

Coronary angiograms, 88, 89, 98

Coronary angioplasty. *See* Angioplasty

Coronary artery bypass graft surgery (CABG): *vs.* angioplasty, 98, 99; development of, 88, 98; efficacy of, 88–90, 99–101; trials of, 89–90, 99–100, 102; as Type II Medical Malpractice, 118

Coronary artery disease: definition of, 88; treatment of, 88–90, 95–101, 183; Type II Medical Malpractice in approach to, 118, 183

Cortisone, 107

"Cost Conundrum, The" (Gawande), 100

Cost of preventing an event (COPE), 198

Cost-plus contracts, 19, 57–58

Costs of health care, 41–70; academic health centers' role in, 47–51; codes in billing for, 65–66; by condition, *42*, 42–43, *43*; development of system for setting, 45–46, 64–68, 200–201; difficulty of data analysis on, 41–42; in Disease Insurance–Health Assurance approach, 195, 198–99; drugs in, 63, 181; *vs.* efficacy, in health-care reform, 179, 182; hospitals' role in, 51–55; institutions behind escalation of, 46, *47*; insurance industry's role in, 55–58; insurance premiums and deductibles in, 69, 191; international comparisons of, 44–45, 58, *59*, 181; interventional *vs.* cognitive specialties in, 46, 68, 218–19; per capita, 5, *44*, 44–45, 58, *59*, 181; as percentage of GDP, 5, 41, 180–81; pharmaceutical industry's role in, 59–63; as reflection of quality and complexity of care, 15; Resource-Based Relative Value Scale for, 67–68, 201; by source of payment, 42–43, *43*; "usual and customary," 45–46, 52, 58, 64–68

Counseling, psychological, 197

COURAGE trial, 99

Courts. *See* Judicial system

CPT. *See* Current Procedural Terminology

Craige, Ernest, *181*

C-reactive protein (CRP), 37, 40

Credentialing, conflicts of interest in, 211

Creosote, 133–34

Crestor, 36–40, 71

CROs. *See* Contract Research Organizations

Cross-sectional studies, 184

CT. *See* Computerized tomography

C282Y genotype, 138

Current Procedural Terminology (CPT), 65, 66, 67, 201

Cutler, David, 178, 179

Cyclobenzaprine, 174

Cymbalta, 175–76

Cypress Bioscience, 174, 176

Dalkon Shield, 103

Data analysis: in comparative effec-

tiveness research, 75–76; of health-care costs, 41–42; of large data sets, 83–84; in trials, 27–29, 75

Daubert Standard of Expert Opinion, 92–95, 100

Daubert v. Merrell Dow Pharmaceuticals, 92, 94

Dawkins, Richard, 158

Death: disease as cause of, 2; international comparison of rates, 44–45; proximate-cause epidemiology on, 124

Death panels, 180

Decision making: clinical interviews in, 196–97; comparative effectiveness research in, 76–77; computerized aids in, 196; efficacy in, 78–90, 185; evidence-based medicine in, 213; randomized controlled trials in, 79–80; reviews of literature in, 213–14. *See also* Clinical judgment

Deductibles, rise of, 69

Deductive reasoning, 123–24

Defibrillators, intracardiac, 105

Denmark, health-care costs in, 181

Depression: drugs in treatment of, 174, 176, 177; placebo effect in, 152

Depressive disease, major, 152

Descartes, René, 168, 169

"Detailing," pharmaceutical, 6–9, *8*

Determinism, linguistic, 169

Detox remedies, 167

Diabetes, cost of treatment of, 42, *42*, *43*

Diabetes, type 1, heritability of, 140

Diabetes, type 2: heritability of, 140; screening for, 135; treatment of, 81, 81n

Diagnoses, for symptoms of unknown origin, 171–72, 174, 177, 209–10

Diagnostic entrepreneurs, 172, 176

Diagnostic radiology, 111–15

Digital rectal exams, 135

DiLorenzo, Thomas J., 36

Dioxin, 134

Direct-to-consumer (DTC) advertising, 33–40; of Crestor, 36–40, 71; efficacy and effectiveness subverted by, 184; of fibromyalgia treatments, 172–73; government regulation of, 9, 33; rise of, 33; spending on, *8*, 33–34, 36

Disability determinations, physicians as gatekeepers in, 208–9

Disclosure, of conflicts of interest, 7–12

Disease(s): absence of, *vs.* good health, 2; definition of, 2; genetics of, 137–42; ICD classification of, 66; natural histories of, 145–46, 152–53; proximate-cause epidemiology in prevention of, 124–25; screening tests in prevention of, 135–36; ubiquity of, 2. *See also specific diseases*

Disease Insurance Account, 194–200

Disease mongering, 172–77

Disease-Related Groups (DRGs), 65–66

Disease-specific foundations, 34–36

Doc-in-the-box movement, 204

Doctors. *See* Physician(s)

Doctor's Dilemma, The (Shaw), 90

Domagk, Gerhard, 60

Double-blind randomized controlled trials. *See* Randomized controlled trials

Downsizing, 130–31

DRGs. *See* Disease-Related Groups

Drugs. *See* Pharmaceutical drugs

Drug trialists, 29, 30, 63

Duisberg, Friedrich Carl, Jr., 60

Duke University Medical Center: Contract Research Organization created by, 24; Institutional Review Boards at, 25; organizational chart of, *18*; pharmacogenetics at, 141–42; ranking of, 23

Duloxetine, 175–76

Durkheim, David Émile, 131

EBM. *See* Evidence-based medicine

Econometrics, 179

Editorials, journal, conflicts of interest in, 11

Education, medical: at academic health centers, 6, 221; clinimetrics centers in, 190; conflicts of interest in, 12–13; at hospitals, 51–52, 54; transition of medical schools into academic health centers, 47–51. *See also* Continuing medical education

Effectiveness: comparative, research on, 74–77; *vs.* efficacy, 74–77, 183–86

Effectiveness Movement, 82

Efficacy, 71–90; common treatments not meeting standard of, 85; design of tests of, 77–78, 184; of devices, 82, 187; in Disease Insurance–Health Assurance approach, 195; *vs.* effectiveness, 74–77, 183–86; in FDA criteria for approval, 73, 82, 92; in health-care reform, 179, 182, 183–86; how to measure, 77–78, 184; in large data sets, 83–84; in observational studies, 145–46, 147, 184; origins of testing for, 73–74; of psychological counseling, 197; in randomized controlled trials, 74–75, 77–78, 184–85; and relative risk reductions, 86–87; reviews of literature on, 213–14; small effects and, 81, 82–83, 185; in treatment decisions, 78–90, 185. *See also specific devices, drugs, and procedures*

Elderly, likelihood of becoming, 126–27

Electronic Health Record (EHR), 65

Eli Lilly and Company, 174, 175

Elion, Gertrude, 25, 61, 190

Elshaug, Adam, 151

EMI, 91

Emotions, in brain, 169

Empirical therapies, 216, 218

Employee Retirement Income Security Act (ERISA) of 1974, 56

Employer(s), in workers' compensation system, 56–57, 69

Employer-based health insurance: cost-plus contracts in, 19, 58; employee contributions to, 69; moral hazards in, 191–92; percent of health-care costs paid by, 42–43, 43; rise in premiums and deductibles for, 69

Employment, and longevity, 129–31

Empowerment, of patients, 206–7

Enablement Fund, 194, 195, 198, 200

End-of-life care, 180

Engel, George, 168

Entrepreneurs, diagnostic, 172, 176

Environmental factors, in genetics, 139

Environmental hazards, public health policy on, 132–34

Environmental Protection Agency (EPA), 132

Epidemiology: history of, 123–24; life-course (social), 125–26; proximate-cause, 123–25; small-effect, 39–40

Épisteme, 163

Epistemology, 71–72

Epstein, Samuel S., 36

Equipose, 87, 89–90

ERISA. *See* Employee Retirement Income Security Act

Ernst, Edzard, 166–67

Estes-Kefauver amendment, 92

Estrogens, 134

Ethics: AMA code of, 64, 166, 200–201; in compassionate use of drugs, 32; in consent forms, 154; in health journalism, 20–21; in insurance industry, 191–93; in scientific process, 12; in screening, 138; in surgical trials, 188. *See also* Conflicts of interest

Europe, pharmaceutical drug costs in, 63, 181. *See also specific countries*

Evaluation/Management Services (E/M), billing codes for, 65

Evidence-based medicine (EBM), 213–14; reviews of literature in, 213–14; rise of, 73, 213; *vs.* sectarian medicine, 157–58. *See also* Efficacy; Randomized controlled trials; Trials

Experiencing the New Genetics (Finkler), 139

Exploratory analysis. *See* Secondary analysis

Facility fees, hospital, 15, 19

Faith healing, 157, 158–60

False positives and negatives, in screening, 136

Federal regulation: of environmental hazards, 132–34; of pharmaceutical marketing, 9, 33; of trials, 25–26, 29–30. *See also* Food and Drug Administration

Fee-for-service health care: in escalation of health-care costs, 46; future of, 200–202; origins of, 46, 64, 200–201. *See also* Medicare

Fee splitting, 46

Feinstein, Alvan, 146

Fetter, Robert, 65

Fiberoptic scopes, 105–6

Fibromyalgia (FM), 171–77; diagnosis of, 171, 172, 209–10; drugs for treatment of, 172–76; as neurologic *vs.* neurotic, 173; symptoms of, 171, 172

Fibromyalgia Story, The (Barker), 172, 177

Fibrositis, 174

Financial conflicts of interest. *See* Conflicts of interest

Finkler, Kaja, 139

Finland, health-care costs in, 181

510(k) clearance pathway for devices, 103–4

Fleming, Alexander, 60

Flexeril, 174

Florey, Howard, 60

Folly of peer review, 101, 217

Food, Drug, and Cosmetic Act, Medical Device Amendments to, 103

Food and Drug Administration (FDA): application process for new drugs, 188–89; conflicts of interest in, 87; devices regulated by, 82, 100, 102–6, 186–87; on direct-to-consumer advertising, 33, 36; on disclosure of conflicts of interest, 10; in Disease Insurance–Health Assurance approach, 195; efficacy in criteria for approval by, 73, 82, 92; expansion of mission of, 73; on fibromyalgia treatment, 172, 174, 175; in health-care reform, 186–87, 188–89; on high blood-sugar treatment, 81; licensing trials for (*See* Trials); on pharmaceutical marketing to physicians, 7; placebo effect and, 151; proposals for reform of, 186; reporting of adverse events to, 31; surgical procedures as exempt from licensing by, 100, 102

Food industry, organic, 134

Ford, Gerald R., 103

Foreign Affairs, 178

Forest Pharmaceuticals, 176

Foucault, Michel, 163, 204–5

Foundation for Integrated Health, 167

France, health-care costs in, 181

Franklin, Benjamin, 149, 157

Freedman, Benjamin, 87

Freedom Trial, 175

Free market: and hospitals, 66–67; and pharmaceutical industry, 63

Free radicals, 110

Free speech, direct-to-consumer advertising as, 9, 33

Frequencies, relative *vs.* absolute, 86–87

Freud, Sigmund, 173

Friedrich Bayer & Co., 60

Friendships, between physicians and patients, 208

Functional magnetic resonance imaging, 173

Futurity.com, 21

Gadamer, Hans-Georg, 199

Galea, Sandro, 126

Gall bladder, removal of, 105–6

Garber, Alan, 151

Gastroenterologists, colonoscopy by, 201

Gatekeeping responsibility: of judges, 93, 94; of physicians, 208–9

Gawande, Atul, 100

Gene signatures, 141, 142

Genetics, 137–42; of disease, 137–42; pharmacogenetics, 140–42; and screening, 137–39

Genomics, 139–42

Genotypes, 137, 138, 139–41

Georgetown University, hospital system of, 23

GERD, 177

Germany, pharmaceutical industry in, 59–60

Gevitz, Norman, 164

Gillings, Dennis, 62–63, 190

Gladwell, Malcolm, 22–23

Glaxo, 61–62

GlaxoSmithKline, 62

God Delusion, The (Dawkins), 158

God Is Not Great (Hitchens), 158

Good manufacturing practices (GMP), 103

Gøtzsche, Peter, 160–61

Government funding: for basic research, 25, 48, 190; for hospitals, 13–14; from NIH, 48–51

Government regulation. *See* Federal regulation; State regulation

Grants, NIH, 48–51

Grassley, Chuck, 6

Greece, poverty and longevity in, 128

Greed: in Medicare fee structure, 45–46; in modern hospital system,

in health-care reform, 191–93, 194; moral hazards in, 191–92; national, in presidential election of 1912, 182, 200; origins and history of, 55–58; rise in premiums and deductibles for, 69; state regulation of, 56; *vs.* workers' compensation system, 55–57

Health insurance companies: business model of, 191–92; cost-plus contracts of, 19, 58; in escalation of health-care costs, 55–58; in health-care reform, 191–93; negotiation of costs with hospitals, 67; number of, per state, 69; percent of health-care costs paid by, 43, *43*; profit of, 19

Health journalism. *See* Journalism, health/medical

Health Maintenance Organizations (HMOs), 46, 58

Health promotion: alcohol consumption and, 119–23; genetics in, 137–42; life-course epidemiology and, 125–26; longevity and, 126–32; proximate-cause epidemiology and, 124–25; public health policy and, 132–36; screening tests in, 135–39

Heart attacks: advances in understanding of, 88; natural history of, 145; quality in treatment of, 183; survival frequency after, 87

Heart disease, cost of treatment of, 42, *42*, *43*

Heart Protection Study Collaborative Group, 40

Height, adult, 134

Hemochromatosis, screening for, 138–39

Hemophilia, 138

Hepatitis C, 140

Heritability, definition of, 139. *See also* Genetics

HIP Health Plan, 46

Hippocrates, 218

Hip replacements, total, 187

Histamine, 61

Historical control, 145–46

Hitchens, Christopher, 158

Hitchings, George, 25, 61, 190

Hodgkin's lymphoma, 111

Hofmann, Felix, 60

Homeopathy, 157, 167

Hôpital Cochin (Paris), 169

Hormone-replacement therapy, 134

Hormones, in environment, 134

Hospital(s), 13–24; billing systems of, 65–67; business model of, 23–24; competition for patients among, 14, 23–24; in escalation of health-care costs, 51–55; facility fees of, 15, 19; fee structures of, 67; for-profit, 15, 19; free market and, 66–67; funding sources for, 13–14, 53–54; in health journalism, 21; history of, 13–15, 51–55; malpractice cases in, 117–18; marketing by, 19–21; medical education at, 51–52, 54; not-for-profit, 15, 19, 52–53; rankings of, 22–23; satellite facilities of, 14, 24; ward services of, 47, 51, 52, 64

Hospital administration: in escalation of health-care costs, 52–53; facility fees to cover cost of, 15; growth of, 14, 52–53; organizational charts for, *16–17, 18*

House officers, 47, 51–52, 54

Housing and Urban Development, Department of (HUD), 142

"How CER Could Pay for Itself" (Elshaug and Garber), 151

Hróbjartsson, Asbjørn, 160–61, 166

Hsiao, William, 67

Human capital, 131

Human Genome Project, 158

Hume, David, 72

Huntington's chorea, 138

Hyaluran, 104, 107
Hypertension, cost of treatment of, 42, *42, 43*
Hypoglycemics, oral, trials of, 81, 81n
Hypotheses, in randomized controlled trials, 27, 74–75

ICD. *See* International Statistical Classification of Diseases and Related Health Problems
"Iceberg of morbidity," 170
ICI, 61
IG Farben, 59–60
Illness: biopsychosocial model of, 168, 169; as in the mind, 168–69, 176, 209–10. *See also* Disease; *specific illnesses*
Imaging procedures, cost of, 42. *See also specific types*
Income: insurance premiums as percent of, 69; and longevity, 126, 128–29; and means-based disparities in health care, 128–29. *See also* Socioeconomic status
Income gap: definition of, 128; and longevity, 128–29
Inductive reasoning, 123–24
Industry, relationships between professionals and, 10, 12
Informed consent: in clinical settings, 96, 154; in randomized controlled trials, 153, 154–55
Injury, back pain as, 129–30
Innovation, in regulation of devices, 104
In-patient nurses, 182
Institute of Medicine, 5, 74, 186
Institutionalization, of conflicts of interest, 12–13, 189–90, 211–12
Institutional Review Boards (IRBs), 25–26
Insurance: malpractice, 67, 117; tort, 193. *See also* Health insurance; Workers' compensation

Insurance Company of North America, 55
International Statistical Classification of Diseases and Related Health Problems (ICD), 66
Internet: continuing medical education on, 220; direct-to-consumer advertising on, 34; health journalism on, 21
Intervention(s): efficacy in decisions about, 78–90, 185; randomized controlled trials as requirement for licensing, 144–45; useless, in health-care reform, 179, 183. *See also specific types*
Interventional cardiology: efficacy of, 88–90, 95–102; rationales for, 100–102; rise of, 97–98; trials of, 89–90, 98–100, 101; Type II Medical Malpractice in, 118. *See also specific procedures*
Interviews, clinical, in Disease Insurance–Health Assurance approach, 196–97
Intracardiac defibrillators, 105
Intrauterine contraceptive devices (IUDs), 103
Invincibility, sense of, 165
Ionizing radiation, 110–15
IRBs. *See* Institutional Review Boards
Iron metabolism, 138
Irritable bowel syndrome (IBS): diagnosis of, 171, 209–10; placebo effect in, 161–64, *162*, 169
Israel, breast cancer in, 137
Ixel, 176

Jansenism, 168–69
Japan: alcohol metabolism in, 140; pharmaceutical drug costs in, 63; workers' compensation claims for backache in, 130
Job satisfaction, and longevity, 129–31

Joffe, Steven, 154

Johnson, Lyndon, 45, 201

Journal(s), medical, conflicts of interest in, 11

Journalism, health/medical: conflicts of interest in, 20–21; demise of, 19–21; ethics in, 20–21; marketing departments as sources of, 21; on medical genetics, 139; university programs in, 20

Journal of Occupational and Environmental Medicine, 93

Journal of Pain, 175

Journal of the American Medical Association, 12–13

Journal of the American Medical Society, 149

Judgment, moral: in conflicts of interest, 8–9; *vs.* conventional judgments, 8. *See also* Clinical judgment

Judicial system: Daubert Standard of Expert Opinion in, 92–95, 100; devices in, 104–5, 186; product-liability suits in, 105, 186; reliability and relevance of scientific information in, 93–94; on sectarian medicine, 166. *See also* Supreme Court; Tort system

Jung, Carl, 173

JUPITER trial, 37–40

Justice, Department of, 54

Kaiser Health, 46

Kandel, Eric, 170

Kansas, health-insurance market in, 69

Kaplan, George, 125

Kaptchuk, Ted, 161–63, 166, 169

"Keyboard for Daubert, A" (Hadler), 93

Klarer, Josef, 60

Knee arthroscopy, 108–9; development of, 108; efficacy of, 108–9; trials of, 108–9

Knee pain: treatment of, 106–9; ubiquity of, 106

Knee replacement, total, observational research on, 76

Knowledge of Man, The (Buber), 210

Koenig, Harold, 159

Kozinski, Alex, 93

Labeling: based on symptoms, 171–72, 209–10; consequences of, 176–77; in fibromyalgia, 171–77

Laboratory of Hygiene, 48

Language of God, The (Collins), 158

Laparoscopy, 105–6

Last Well Person, The (Hadler), 1

Leaders, thought, 30, 63, 189, 221

Leadership, and professionalism, 211

Lederle, 36

Lehrer, Jonah, 152

Leukemia, 111, 132, 133

Liberty Mutual, 56

Licensing trials. *See* Trials

Life-course epidemiology, 125–26

Life expectancy, socioeconomic status and, 126, 128. *See also* Longevity

Life problems, and back pain, 130

Lincoln, Abraham, 179

Lind, James, 73

Linguistic determinism, 169

Lipid abnormalities, cost of treatment of, 42, *42*, *43*

Literature, medical: competitive nature of science and, 12; conflicts of interest in, 10–12; reviews of, 213–14

Lobbying, of Congress, 6, 180, 201

Longevity, 126–32; alcohol consumption and, 119–23, *122*; historical changes to rates of, 126–27, *127*, 134; life-course epidemiology on, 125–26; psychosocial challenges and, *122*, 123, 129–32; social cohesiveness and, 131–32, 143; socioeconomic status and, 121, *122*, 123, 126–29

Lottery mentality, 79–82

Louis XVI (king of France), 149

Low back pain. *See* Back pain
Löwig, Karl, 59
Lung cancer, treatment of, 78–80
Lupus erythematosus, systemic, heritability of, 140
Lymphoma, 111
Lyrica, 174–75

Magnetic resonance imaging (MRI): of cancer, 146; *vs.* CT imaging, 115; of fibromyalgia, 173; for knee pain, 107; static field in, 109
Magnetic therapies, 149, 157
Malpractice. *See* Medical malpractice
Mammography: effectiveness of, 135, 136, 137; genetics and, 137–38; ionizing radiation in, 112, *113*; Preventive Services Task Force on, 192
Marine Hospital Service, 48
Marketing: and health journalism, 19–21; by hospitals and academic health centers, 19–21, 221; physician rankings as, 22–23. *See also* Direct-to-consumer advertising; Pharmaceutical marketing
Marmot, Sir Michael, 125
Marvels, medical, 72–73
Marx, Karl, 131
Massachusetts, pharmaceutical marketing in, 9
Massachusetts General Hospital, 51–52
MASS-II trial, 99–100
Mastectomies, 137
May & Baker, Ltd., 60
Mayo Clinic, 46
Media coverage. *See* Journalism, health/medical
Medicaid, nomenclature for billing in, 65
Medical Device Amendments to Food, Drug, and Cosmetic Act, 103
Medical education. *See* Education, medical

Medical Expenditure Panel Survey (MEPS), 41–43, *42, 43*
Medicalization, 170–72; of genetics, 139; and health-care reform, 180
Medical literature. *See* Literature, medical
Medical malpractice: in hospitals, 117–18; insurance, 67, 117; Type I, 115–18; Type II, 118, 183
Medical pluralism, 165
Medical research. *See* Research, medical
Medical Research Council (MRC), 25, 190
Medical schools, transition into academic health centers, 47–51. *See also* Education, medical
Medicare: in escalation of health-care costs, 45–46, 52–54; establishment of, 45, 201; facility fees in, 15; fee structure of, 45–46, 53–54, 201; growth in complexity of, 53; nomenclature for billing in, 65; private sector in administration of, 58; rise of cost of, 181; vertebroplasties covered by, 151
Medicine: art of, 205–7; contemporary institution of, 211–12
Medicine, Religion, and Health (Koenig), 159
Medtronic, 104–5
Melanoma, 110
Menarche, age of, 134
Menopause, age at, 134
Mental disorders, cost of treatment of, *42, 43*
MEPS. *See* Medical Expenditure Panel Survey
Merck, 174
Merck Institute, 25
Mesmer, Franz Anton, 149, 157
Mesmerism, 149, 157
Metabolic syndrome, 125–26

Metaphysical belief systems, 157–59

Metzger, Henry, 49

Microecology, 127–28

Mietzsch, Fritz, 60

Miles Laboratories, 60

Mill, John Stuart, 72

Miller, Franklin, 161–63, 166

Milnacipran, 176

Mind: in mind-body duality, 163, 167–70; in placebo effect, 160–64, 169; symptoms as being in the, 168–69, 176, 209–10

Minnesota: pharmaceutical marketing in, 9; regulation of devices in, 105

"Minor" medical treatments, in retail store clinics, 204

Misery, medicalization of, 170–72

Money. *See* Costs of health care; Profit

Mor, Gil, 141

Moral judgments: in conflicts of interest, 8–9; *vs.* conventional judgments, 8

"Morbidity, iceberg of," 170

"Morbidity and Mortality Conferences," 217

Morse, Robert, 22

Mortality: alcohol consumption and, 121–23, *122*; psychosocial and socioeconomic influences on, 126–32. *See also* Death

MRC. *See* Medical Research Council

MRI. *See* Magnetic resonance imaging

Municipal bonds, 14, 53

Muscle relaxants, 174

Muscular dystrophy, 138

National Academy of Social Insurance, 179

National Cancer Institute, 21, 35

National Center for Health Statistics, 66

National health insurance, in presidential election of 1912, 182, 200

National Heart Act of 1948, 48

National Institute of Arthritis and Metabolic Diseases, 49

National Institutes of Health (NIH), 48–51; budget of, 48; cardiology trials sponsored by, 89, 99; Clinical Center of, 48, 49; on conflicts of interest, 11; disease-specific advocacy groups and, 35; extramural research programs of, 48, 49–50; history of, 48–49; indirect costs paid to institutions by, 50–51; influence on medical field, 48–51; intramural research programs of, 48–49; primary research at, 25, 48, 190; religious views at, 158; staff of, 49

National steering committee, for randomized controlled trials, 190, 196, 197

Natural histories, of diseases, 145–46, 152–53

Nature, 141

NDAs. *See* New drug applications

Neck pain, 147

"Negative Income Tax" experiment, 142–43

Neuroimaging, 169–70

Neurosis: evolution of term, 173; and fibromyalgia, 173

New drug applications (NDAs), Contract Research Organizations in, 188–89

New England Journal of Medicine: conflicts of interest in, 11; equipose in, 87; placebo effect in, 151, 161; results of JUPITER trial in, 37; results of STICH trial in, 90

New Jersey, billing based on Disease-Related Groups in, 65

Newton, Sir Isaac, 72

New Yorker, 152, 166

New Zealand, direct-to-consumer advertising in, 33

NIH. *See* National Institutes of Health

Nixon, Richard, 35, 142

NNH. *See* Number needed to harm

NNT. *See* Number needed to treat

Nobel Prizes, 25, 60, 61, 111, 131, 170, 190

Nocebo, 163–65

Nonagenarians, historical changes to rates of, 127, *127*

Nordic Cochrane Centre, 160–61

North Carolina Memorial Hospital, history of, 13–14, *181. See also* UNC Hospitals

Not-for-profit hospitals, 15, 19, 52–53

Novant, 15

Nuclear disasters, 109, 111

Number needed to harm (NNH), 185

Number needed to treat (NNT): definition of, 77–78; in Disease Insurance–Health Assurance approach, 195–96, 198; and efficacy, 77–78, 82, 85; in health-care reform, 184–85, 195–96, 198; maximum acceptable number for, 78, 82, 85, 195

Nurse practitioners, colonoscopy by, 201

Nurses, in-patient, 182

Nutrition: in adult height, 134; in poverty and longevity, 129

OAT trial, 99

Obama, Barack, 74, 179, 182

Obesity, changes in perception of, 2

Observational studies: determination of efficacy in, 145–46, 147, 184; on devices, 103; on environmental hazards, 133; limitations of, 76, 145–46, 184; *vs.* randomized controlled trials, 145–46, 184; subjectivity in reporting of symptoms in, 147; on surgical procedures, 108; types of, 184

Octogenarians, historical changes to rates of, 126–27, *127*

Odds ratio, 123

Off-label use of pharmaceutical drugs, 30–33, 216

Of Regimen of Health (Bacon), 158

Ohio, workers' compensation in, 56

Oil industry, 132–33

Omnibus Budget Reconciliation Act of 1989, 67

Oncology: disease foundations dedicated to, 35–36; off-label use of drugs in, 31; radiation, 112. *See also* Cancer

Oncotype DX, 141

"Order of Things, The" (Gladwell), 22–23

Oregon, health-insurance market in, 69

Organic food industry, 134

Organizational policies: on pharmaceutical marketing to physicians, 6; on pharmaceutical marketing to practitioners, 7

Orgasms, changes in perception of, 2

Orszag, Peter, 178, 179, 180

Osteoarthritis, cost of treatment of, 42, *42, 43*

Osteopathy, 157

Osteoporotic compression fractures, treatment of, 151–52

Other Healers (Gevitz), 164

Ovarian cancer, genetics of, 137, 141

OvaSure test, 141

Pacemakers, 103

Pain: placebo and, 149–52, 156; ubiquity of, 199. *See also specific types*

Pap smears, 135

Pascal, Blaise, 168–69

Patents, on pharmaceutical drugs, 63

Paternalism, in physician-patient interactions, 204–5, 206

Patients: competition for, 14, 23–24; as consumers, 91; empowerment of, 206–7; physician relationship with

(*See* Physician-patient relationship); physician responsibility to, *vs.* industrial success, 10; in trials (*See* Trials); as units of care, 212

PBBs, 134

PCBs, 134

Peer learning, interactive, 216–17, 220

Peer review: in clinical judgment, 215–17; competitive nature of science and, 12; conflicts of interest in, 11, 211; folly of, 101, 217; limitations of, 216–17; of off-label use of drugs, 31

Penicillin, 60

Pentagon, 19, 57

Pentecostalism, 157

Peppercorn, Jeffrey, 154

PET. *See* Positron emission tomography

Petrochemicals, 132–33

Pfisterer, Matthias, 99

Pfizer Pharmaceutical, 172–73, 174–75

Phantom limbs, 168

Pharmaceutical devices, 91–118; classification system for, 103; conflicts of interest in literature on, 11–12; conflicts of interest in marketing of, 6–10; criteria for approval of, 82; definition of, 104; efficacy of, 82, 187; FDA regulation of, 82, 100, 102–6, 186–87; in health-care reform, 186–88; state regulation of, 104–5; tort immunity for, 96, 186; trials of, 187. *See also specific devices*

Pharmaceutical drugs: conflicts of interest in literature on, 11–12; conflicts of interest in marketing of, 6–10; criteria for approval of, 73, 82; development process for new, 24–25; direct-to-consumer advertising of, 9, 33–34; for fibromyalgia, 172–76; genetics in metabolism of, 140–42; in health-care reform, 183–86, 188–90; international differences

in costs of, 63, 181; off-label and compassionate use of, 30–33, 216; *vs.* placebo, effects of, 150–53; and rise of epidemiology, 123–24; samples of, 6–9. *See also* Trials; *specific drugs*

Pharmaceutical industry: business model of, 189; in escalation of health-care costs, 59–63; history of, 59–63; in-house research in, 25, 60–62, 190; mergers in, 62; outsourcing of novel research by, 25, 62; outsourcing of trials by, 24–30, 62–63, 189–90; price setting in, 63

Pharmaceutical marketing, to consumers. *See* Direct-to-consumer advertising

Pharmaceutical marketing, to physicians: conflict of interest in, 6–10, 211; efficacy and effectiveness subverted by, 184; government regulation of, 9; methods of, 6–7; organizational policies on, 6, 7; through seed trials, 30; spending on, 7, *8*

Pharmacogenetics, 140–42

Phase I trials, 26

Phase II trials, 26, 32–33

Phase III trials, 26–29, 32–33

Phase IV trials, 32

Phenotypes, 139

Philosophers, physicians as, 72, 207

Philosopher's stone, 72–73, 74

Phocomelia, 92

Phthalates, 134

Physician(s): art of medicine and, 205–7; disclosure of conflicts of interest by, 7–12; as gatekeepers, 208–9; pharmaceutical marketing to, 6–10, 30, 184, 211; as philosophers, 72, 207; public calling of, 64, 200, 203; rankings of, 22–23; responsibility for industrial success *vs.* patient benefit, 10; in setting of fee structure,

45–46; specializing in procedures *vs.* diagnosis/management, 46

Physician-patient relationship: art of medicine in, 205–7; clinical judgment in, 207–12; as collaboration, 204–5, 207–8; paternalism in, 204–5, 206; trust in, 207–8, 209–10. *See also* Decision making

"Placebo Effect Studies Are Susceptible to Response Bias and to Other Types of Biases" (Kaptchuk, Miller, and Hróbjartsson), 166

Placebos, 148–56; effects of, without deceptive protocols, 161–63; *vs.* faith healing, 160; harm caused by, 163–65; history of use of, 148–50; origins of term, 163; for pain, 149; in randomized controlled trials, 26, 27, 148–56, 160–63; role of mind in, 160–64, 169; in sectarian medicine, 157, 164–65, 167; in surgical trials, 188

Plaques: definition of, 88; treatment of, 88, 89

Plastics, 134

Pluralism, medical, 165

Pollution. *See* Environmental hazards

Polygenic traits, 139–40

Popper, Karl, 72

Portable Atheist, The (Hitchens), 158

Positron emission tomography (PET), 115, 146

Potti, Anil, 142

Poverty: definitions of, 128; longevity and, 126, 128–29; social cohesiveness and, 142–43. *See also* Socioeconomic status

Power considerations, in randomized controlled trials, 75

"Powerful Placebo, The" (Beecher), 149

Practitioners. *See* Physician(s)

Pregabalin, 174–75

Premiums, rise of, 69

Presidential election of 1912, health-care reform in, 182, 200

Preventive Services Task Force, U.S.: on efficacy, 185; screening recommendations of, 138–39, 192

Prevent-treat-cure strategy, 3

Prices. *See* Costs

Priesthood, medical, 204–5

Primary hypotheses, 75

Private sector: medical research in, 12, 190; in Medicare administration, 58. *See also* Contract Research Organizations

Procedures. *See* Surgical procedures

Product-liability suits, 105, 186

Professionalism: clinical judgment in, 207–10; in contemporary institution of medicine, 211–12; timeliness in, 208

Profit: of academic health centers, 6, 15; of health insurance companies, 19; in pharmaceutical industry, 190; in workers' compensation, 56–57, 192

Progressive Party, 182, 200

Prontisil, 60

Proof, absence of, 85

Propanolol, 61

Proprietary hospitals, 51, 52

Prostate cancer, screening for, 81, 135, 136, 192

Prostate-specific antigen (PSA), 81, 135, 136, 192

Proteomics, 141

Proximate-cause epidemiology, 123–25

PSA. *See* Prostate-specific antigen

Psychoimmunology, 129

Psychological counseling, 197

Psychosocial challenges: and alcohol consumption, *122*, 123; in biopsycho-social model of illness, 168; and cardiovascular disease, 125–26; and longevity, *122*, 123, 129–32; and symptoms, 147–48

Psychotropic agents, 152
Puberty, age of, 134
Public calling, medicine as, 64, 200, 203
Public Health Hospital system, 48
Public health policy, 132–36; on environmental hazards, 132–34; on screening tests, 135–36
Public Health Service, 48, 49
Public sector: medical research in, 12, 190; randomized controlled trials as responsibility of, 190
Pulmonary diseases, cost of treatment of, *42, 43*
Purchasing power, poverty as measure of, 128

Quackery, 101, 166
Quality: as goal of health-care reform, 182–83; measures of, in physician rankings, 22
Quintiles Transnational, 24, 63, 189, 190

Radiation: normal exposure to, 110–11; types of, 109–10
Radiation hormesis, 111
Radiation therapy, 111
Radiobiology, 109–15
Radiology, diagnostic, 111–15
Radiomimetic drugs, 111
Rand, Ayn, 132
Randomization errors, 82–83
Randomized controlled trials (RCTs), 26–30; analysis of data from, 27–29, 75; average responses in, 79–80; clinically meaningful outcomes of, 77–78; *vs.* comparative effectiveness research, 74–75; in decision making, 79–81; design of, 26–27, 74–75, 77–78; development of methodology of, 73; in Disease Insurance–Health Assurance approach, 195–96; double-blind protocol for, 26–27, 149; effi-

cacy tested in, 74–75, 77–78, 83–84, 184–85; equipose in, 87; in health-care reform, 184–91, 195–96; importance of, 73–74, 144; informed consent in, 153, 154–55; of interventions, as requirement for licensing, 144–45; in judicial system, 93; limitations of, 75; number of subjects needed for, 27–28, 75; *vs.* observational studies, 145–46, 184; and off-label and compassionate use of drugs, 30–33; origins of, 73; pharmaceutical firms' outsourcing of, 24–30, 62–63, 189–90; placebos in, 26, 27, 148–56, 160–63; preconceptions and expectations of subjects in, 153–56; of psychological counseling, 197; as public-sector responsibility, 190; randomization errors in, 82–83; recruitment of subjects for, 29–30, 153–54, 197; of sectarian medicine, 164, 167; of surgical procedures, 187–88; time frames of, 83–84; of two active drugs, 148, 150; of two devices or procedures, 187. *See also* Placebos; *specific drugs*
Ranitidine, 62
Rankings, of hospitals and physicians, 22–23
Ransdell Act of 1930, 48
Ransohoff, David, 141
Rationality: in health-care system, 180–82; in medical decision making, 78, 80
Rationing of health care, 139, 180
RBRVS. *See* Resource-Based Relative Value Scale
RBRVS Update Committee (RUC), 67–68, 201
RCTs. *See* Randomized controlled trials
Realpolitik, 211–12
Records, medical, coding in, 65
Reductionism, in epidemiology, 124
Reform. *See* Health-care reform

157, 164–65, 167; trials of, 157, 164, 167; wellness in, 164–65

Seed trials, 30, 63

Self-insured employers: health insurance of, 58; workers' compensation system of, 56–57

Sensitivity, of screening tests, 136

Sham-surgery trials: of coronary artery bypass graft surgery, 102; ethics of, 188; of knee arthroscopy, 108–9; of vertebral fractures, 151

Shaw, George Bernard, 90

Sherman Antitrust Act, 166

Sick leave, 130

Sigmoidoscopy, 135, 136

Siler, Anne, 175

Single-payer insurance system, 192

Skin cancer, 110

Sliding scale, 64, 201

Small effectology, 83, 185, 189

Small effects: of environmental hazards, 133; in trials, 39–40, 81, 82–83, 185, 189

Smith Kline and French (SKF), 61, 62

Social capital, 130, 131, 143

Social cohesiveness: and effects of poverty, 142–43; and job satisfaction, 130; and longevity, 131–32, 143

Social construction, of well-being, 2

Social epidemiology, 125–26

Society, definition of, 131

Society of Professional Journalism, 20

Socioeconomic status: and alcohol consumption, 121, *122*, 123; and cardiovascular disease, 125–26; and longevity, 121, *122*, 123, 126–29; and means-based disparities in health care, 128–29

Soft outcomes, 146–56; in observational studies, 146, 147; placebos and, 148–56; in trials, 28, 30, 146, 148–56, 195–96

Somatoform disorders, 173, 210

Soul, 168–69

South Korea, health-care costs in, 181

Specializations, medical: in fee structures, 67–68, 218–19; rise of, 46, 47, 49

Specificity, of screening tests, 136

Spinal manipulation, 155–56

Spine surgery: trials of, 187–88; as Type II Medical Malpractice, 118

Squamous cell carcinoma, 110

Stabbed in the Back (Hadler), 1, 56, 57, 118, 129, 131, 148, 152, 160, 209, 210

Staffing, redundancies in, 182

Stage migration, 146

State regulation: of billing based on Disease-Related Groups, 65–66; of devices, 104–5; of direct-to-consumer advertising, 9; in Disease Insurance–Health Assurance approach, 194–200; of health insurance, 56; of workers' compensation, 55–57

Statins, efficacy of, 80–81. *See also* Crestor

Statistical significance: definition of, 83; in randomized controlled trials, 75, 77, 83, 84, 184–85; of relative frequencies, 86–87

Steering committee, for randomized controlled trials, 190, 196, 197

Stents: development of, 98; efficacy of, 96–101; trials of, 98–99; as Type II Medical Malpractice, 118

Sterling Products, 60

STICH trial, 90

Streptomycin, 61

Stress, of poverty, 129

Subjectivity, in reporting of symptoms, 147–48

Sulfonamidochrysoidine, 60

Sulphapyridine, 60

Supreme Court, U.S.: Daubert Standard of, 92–95, 100; on device manufacturers, 105, 186; on pharmaceutical marketing to consumers, 9; on sectarian medicine, 166; on workers' compensation, 55

Surgical procedures: cost of, 42; as exempt from FDA licensing, 100, 102; in health-care reform, 186–88; history of advances in, 218; trials of, 187–88. *See also specific procedures*

Surrogate measures of trials, 28, 75

Symptoms, 147–48; absence of, *vs.* good health, 2; labeling based on, 171–72, 209–10; measuring relief of, 147–48; medicalization of, 170–72; as in the mind, 168–69, 176, 209–10; placebo effect in, 152–53, 160–63; psychosocial context of, 147–48; subjectivity in reporting of, 147–48; trials of surgical interventions for, 188; ubiquity of, 2, 170; of unknown origin, 171–72, 174, 177, 209–10; in wellness, 170–72

Tagamet, 61

Talk therapy, 197

Tax exemptions: for employer-based health insurance, 43; for workers' compensation, 57

Temporomandibular joint syndrome (TMJ), 209–10

Texas, workers' compensation in, 56

Thalidomide, 73, 92

Theories, testing of, 71–74

Thompson, John, 65

Thought leaders, 30, 63, 189, 221

Toasting, 119–20

Tort system, 115–18; device manufacturers in, 105, 186; in health-care reform, 193; immunity in, 56, 96, 105, 186

Total knee replacement (TKR), observational research on, 76

Toxicity, in Phase II trials, 33

Toxins, environmental, 132–34

Translational research, 10, 24, 83

Transparency: in billing and costs, 67, 68; in health insurance, 58; in modern hospital system, 15

Trauma-related disorders, cost of treatment of, 42, *42, 43*

Treatments, efficacy in decisions about, 78–90, 185. *See also specific types*

Trial and error, in medicine, 73

Trialists, drug, 29, 30, 63

Trials, 24–30; conflicts of interest in, 24–33, 36–40, 63; data analysis in, 27–29; for drugs *vs.* devices, 24; Institutional Review Boards on, 25–26; number of subjects needed for, 27–28; and off-label and compassionate use of drugs, 30–33; Phase I, 26; Phase II, 26, 32–33; Phase III, 26–29, 32–33; Phase IV, 32; recruitment of subjects for, 24, 26, 29–30; reviews of literature on, 213–14. *See also* Randomized controlled trials; *specific drugs*

Trick or Treat (Ernst), 167

Tricyclic antidepressants, 174

Truman, Harry, 48

Trust, in physician-patient relationship, 207–8, 209–10

"Truth Wears Off, The" (Lehrer), 152

Tuberculosis, 140, 145

Tumor-specific chemotherapeutic agents, 140–41

Ultraviolet radiation, 110

UNC Hospitals: administration of, 14, *16–17*; history of, 13–14; marketing of, 19; mission of, 14

Under the Medical Gaze (Greenhalgh), 176–77

United Kingdom, Medical Research Council in, 25, 190

U.S. News & World Report, 22–23

University of Louisville, hospital system of, 23

University of Missouri, health journalism at, 20

University of North Carolina: health journalism at, 20; medical school of, *181*; ranking of, 23

University of Pennsylvania, hospital system of, 15, 23

U-shaped curves, 120–23, 124

"Usual and customary" fees: and cost-plus provisions, 58; in escalation of health-care costs, 45–46, 64–68; in hospitals, 52; new approach to replace, 67–68; origins of, 45–46, 64

Validity, *vs.* reliability, 94

Vane, John, 25, 61

Verbrugge, Lois, 170

Vertebral fractures, treatment of, 151–52, 192

Vertebroplasties, 151–52, 192

Veterans Administration, 32, 89, 108

Veterans Affairs Diabetes Trial, 81n

Viagra, 31

Vietnam War, 49

Waksman, Selman, 25, 60–61

Walmart, 15

Ward services, 47, 51, 52, 64

War on Cancer, 35

Washington, workers' compensation in, 56

Weber, Max, 131

Web seminars, 220

Websites. *See* Internet

Well-being: perceptions of, 2; social construction of, 2

Wellcome Institute, 25

Wellcome Research Laboratories, 61

Wellness: experience of symptoms in, 170–72; in sectarian medicine, 164–65

"West of Scotland" Trial, 80n

West Virginia, health-insurance market in, 69

White, Paul Dudley, *181*

Wilk, Chester A., 166

Wilkinson, Richard, 125

Will Rogers Effect, 146

Wilson, Woodrow, 182

Work, and longevity, 129–31

Workers' compensation: claims for back pain under, 57, 129–30; current system of, 55–57, 69, 192–93; in health-care reform, 191, 192–93; job satisfaction and, 129–30

Workplace safety, 131

World Health Organization (WHO), 44, 66

Worried Sick (Hadler), 1, 81n, 124, 210

Wulff, Katherine, 151

Xenoestrogens, 134

X-rays: of cancer, 146; ionizing radiation from, 110, 111–13, *113*

Zantac, 62

Zinc, 155

Zorprin, 62

Lamar Cecil, *Wilhelm II: Prince and Emperor, 1859–1900* (1989).

Carolyn Merchant, *Ecological Revolutions: Nature, Gender, and Science in New England* (1989).

Gladys Engel Lang and Kurt Lang, *Etched in Memory: The Building and Survival of Artistic Reputation* (1990).

Howard Jones, *Union in Peril: The Crisis over British Intervention in the Civil War* (1992).

Robert L. Dorman, *Revolt of the Provinces: The Regionalist Movement in America* (1993).

Peter N. Stearns, *Meaning Over Memory: Recasting the Teaching of Culture and History* (1993).

Thomas Wolfe, *The Good Child's River*, edited with an introduction by Suzanne Stutman (1994).

Warren A. Nord, *Religion and American Education: Rethinking a National Dilemma* (1995).

David E. Whisnant, *Rascally Signs in Sacred Places: The Politics of Culture in Nicaragua* (1995).

Lamar Cecil, *Wilhelm II: Emperor and Exile, 1900–1941* (1996).

Jonathan Hartlyn, *The Struggle for Democratic Politics in the Dominican Republic* (1998).

Louis A. Pérez Jr., *On Becoming Cuban: Identity, Nationality, and Culture* (1999).

Yaakov Ariel, *Evangelizing the Chosen People: Missions to the Jews in America, 1880–2000* (2000).

Philip F. Gura, *C. F. Martin and His Guitars, 1796–1873* (2003).

Louis A. Pérez Jr., *To Die in Cuba: Suicide and Society* (2005).

Peter Filene, *The Joy of Teaching: A Practical Guide for New College Instructors* (2005).

John Charles Boger and Gary Orfield, eds., *School Resegregation: Must the South Turn Back?* (2005).

Jock Lauterer, *Community Journalism: Relentlessly Local* (2006).

Michael H. Hunt, *The American Ascendancy: How the United States Gained and Wielded Global Dominance* (2007).

Michael Lienesch, *In the Beginning: Fundamentalism, the Scopes Trial, and the Making of the Antievolution Movement* (2007).

Eric L. Muller, *American Inquisition: The Hunt for Japanese American Disloyalty in World War II* (2007).

John McGowan, *American Liberalism: An Interpretation for Our Time* (2007).

Nortin M. Hadler, M.D., *Worried Sick: A Prescription for Health in an Overtreated America* (2008).

William Ferris, *Give My Poor Heart Ease: Voices of the Mississippi Blues* (2009).

Colin A. Palmer, *Cheddi Jagan and the Politics of Power: British Guiana's Struggle for Independence* (2010).

W. Fitzhugh Brundage, *Beyond Blackface: African Americans and the Creation of American Mass Culture, 1890–1930* (2011).

Michael H. Hunt and Steven I. Levine, *Arc of Empire: America's Wars in Asia from the Philippines to Vietnam* (2012).

Nortin M. Hadler, M.D., *The Citizen Patient: Reforming Health Care for the Sake of the Patient, Not the System* (2013).